"Dr. John McDougall turns the toxic stew of American diets into vegetable garden broth."
—*Sonoma Business News*

"Scientific understanding of good nutrition is but one step; putting it into practice is quite another. John and Mary McDougall have done both."
—T. Colin Campbell, Cornell University, and Karen Campbell

"The McDougalls' work is wonderful . . . a gateway to greater health and better living."
—John and Deo Robbins, founders of EarthSave

"Let go of the old habits and live a full, rich life. Try eight- to ten-percent fat and watch a new life blossom."
—*California Press Democrat*

"Dr. John McDougall pushes lifestyle changes that keep your belly full and your tummy flat."   —*Niagara Gazette*

"More compelling reasons for health-conscious individuals to switch to a high-carbohydrate diet."
—*Richmond Mirror*

JOHN A. McDOUGALL, M.D., is a board-certified internist who created and runs the nationally recognized McDougall Program at St. Helena Hospital in California. MARY McDOUGALL, a nurse, teaches with John McDougall and writes the recipes for their books. They are the authors of *The New McDougall Cookbook* (Dutton), *The McDougall Program* (Plume), and several other best-selling books. They live in northern California.

Also by John A. McDougall, M.D.

THE McDOUGALL PLAN

THE McDOUGALL PROGRAM: 12 DAYS TO DYNAMIC HEALTH

THE NEW McDOUGALL COOKBOOK
(with Mary McDougall)

McDougall's Medicine: A Challenging Second Opinion

The McDougall Health-Supporting Cookbooks,
Volumes I and II

THE McDougall Program for Maximum Weight Loss

John A. McDougall, M.D.
Recipes by Mary McDougall

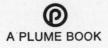

A PLUME BOOK

PLUME
Published by the Penguin Group
Penguin Books USA Inc., 375 Hudson Street, New York, New York 10014, U.S.A.
Penguin Books Ltd, 27 Wrights Lane, London W8 5TZ, England
Penguin Books Australia Ltd, Ringwood, Victoria, Australia
Penguin Books Canada Ltd, 10 Alcorn Avenue, Toronto, Ontario, Canada M4V 3B2
Penguin Books (N.Z.) Ltd, 182–190 Wairau Road, Auckland 10, New Zealand

Penguin Books Ltd, Registered Offices: Harmondsworth, Middlesex, England

Published by Plume, an imprint of Dutton Signet,
a division of Penguin Books USA Inc.
Previously published in a Dutton edition.

First Plume Printing, April, 1995

15 16 17 18 19 20

Copyright © John A. McDougall, 1994
All rights reserved

Calculations for nutritional values were made from:
Pennington, J. *Food Values of Portions Commonly Used*. 14th and 15th Editions,
Harper & Row, New York, 1985 and 1989.
Nutritive Value of American Foods in Common Units, Agriculture Handbook No. 456.
Agriculture Research Services, U.S. Department of Agriculture, 1975.
Composition of Foods. Agriculture Handbook No. 8. U.S. Department of Agriculture,
Science and Education Administration. Revised 1976 to 1980.

℗ REGISTERED TRADEMARK—MARCA REGISTRADA

The Library of Congress has catalogued the Dutton edition as follows:
McDougall, John A.
The McDougall program for maximum weight loss / John A. McDougall;
recipes by Mary McDougall.
p.   cm.
ISBN 0-525-93678-5 (hc.)
ISBN 0-452-27380-3 (pbk.)
1. Reducing diets—Recipes.   2. Complex carbohydrate diet—
Recipes.   3. Low-fat diet—Recipes.   I. McDougall, Mary A. (Mary
Ann)   II. Title.
RM 222.2.M4344   1994
613.2′5—dc20   93–39898
                                                          CIP

Printed in the United States of America
Original hardcover design by Eve L. Kirch

BOOKS ARE AVAILABLE AT QUANTITY DISCOUNTS WHEN USED TO PROMOTE PRODUCTS
OR SERVICES. FOR INFORMATION PLEASE WRITE TO PREMIUM MARKETING DIVISION,
PENGUIN BOOKS USA INC., 375 HUDSON STREET, NEW YORK, NEW YORK 10014.

To those who suffer needlessly in order to look great

ACKNOWLEDGMENTS

Our gratitude and thanks to:

Tom Monte for polishing my rough manuscript into a real book. My office staff—Heather McDougall, Linda Lessard, and Louise Burk—who helped me gather information for this work. The University of California, Davis, Medical Library, which provided the scientific information in this book that supports a simple observation: People who follow a starch-based diet are thin and healthy, and those who feast from a table fit for kings and queens are fat and sickly.

Both Mary and I want to thank our friends, patients, and readers of our books and newsletter for all the valuable lessons you have taught us over the years, and the health and recipe ideas many of you have contributed. A special thanks to the hundreds of people who shared with us their successful experiences on the McDougall Program, as well as the failures they have had in the past on other programs. Unfortunately, only a few stories could be included.

If you have a question or an idea you would like to share, please write:

The McDougalls
P.O. Box 14039
Santa Rosa, CA 95402

CONTENTS

CHAPTER 1

Never Be Hungry or Fat Again

Imagine having to decide between being physically attractive or being able to eat. Well, that's the conflict facing most people every day. You are told by countless diet doctors and weight-loss gurus that in order to lose weight, you must control one of your most basic and powerful instincts: hunger.

That advice, however, is the surest path to yet another failed weight-loss program. The desire to appreciate your body and make it beautiful is one of the most natural and wonderful urges in life. And indeed, everyone can improve his or her looks; all of us can radiate our own natural beauty. Even more fundamental is the urge to eat, which, after all, keeps us alive. The notion that these two very basic instincts are in opposition is not only wrong, but downright self-destructive. It is this cultural delusion that promotes guilt and frustration, and—as we will see later—helps to keep people overweight.

The truth is, you cannot maintain a diet that keeps you hungry. One of your most powerful instincts is to avoid starvation. The only diet that can be sustained—by anyone—is a diet that allows you to eat until you are full and, at the same time, promotes weight loss and good health.

I know what you're thinking: That sounds too good to be true. You've been trained by so many bad experiences with failed diets to think that weight loss can be accomplished only by food deprivation, in one form or another. The most common form of fasting is counting calories and, of course, limiting them. But you have also learned that you can't starve forever. Eventually, you've got to break out of the straitjacket of hunger and go back to your habitual way of eating. Then you regain the weight you lost through great suffering, and in less than half the time it took you to lose it.

The exceedingly difficult task of subduing hunger (it may well be impossible) causes many people to give up any hope of normalizing their weight. When they read my books or hear me say that they can lose weight and eat all they want, they can't believe their eyes or ears.

But that's exactly what you do on the McDougall Program for Maximum Weight Loss. On my diet, you are encouraged to eat as much as you want, as often as you want. There is no calorie-counting or complicated calculations. You can forget portion control forever. In fact, you are strongly encouraged to eat from an incredible variety of delicious foods. Meanwhile, you will lose weight. You will feel great and in no time will look great, too. That's the experience of hundreds of thousands of people who have followed my program.

Misinformation Has Got You in Trouble

Throughout the course of this book, I'll be dispelling misinformation and incorrect beliefs that have kept you from reducing your weight and keeping it off. It's easy to have these misconceptions, many of which are reinforced almost daily by the popular media. When misinformation is repeated over and over again, we eventually accept it as truth. Let me give you an example of just such a phenomenon: Through the 1950s, 1960s, and 1970s, we were trained to believe that beef was the very best food we could be eating. Now science is proving just the opposite. Today, equally erroneous beliefs are being drummed into us. One of them is that olive oil is a health food. In fact, I'll bet you think of olive oil as good for you and sugar as poisonous. But when it comes to losing weight, you're wrong.

All oils are 100 percent fat; they are merely liquid at room temperature. Like all other forms of fat, olive oil contains nine calories per gram, while sugar has only four calories per gram. That means that olive oil contains more than twice the calories per serving than sugar does. In fact, fat is the most calorically dense food in nature.

When we look at what your body does with olive oil and sugar, we find that olive oil is even more harmful to your weight-loss program because it is more easily stored as fat than is sugar. The body treats all fats as "reserve fuel," which means they are stored for the day when you have insufficient carbohydrates to eat. Those fats are kept in your adipose tissues, found mostly under the surface of your skin and surrounding your organs. In other words, that fat makes you fatter. On the other hand, excess sugar is stored invisibly in your muscles and liver as glycogen, or burned off as heat. As we will explore in greater detail later on, sugar is not readily converted to fat in your body, and consequently doesn't affect your weight or appearance.

Moreover, sugar tends to satisfy the appetite by filling the body's carbohydrate needs and replenishing glycogen stores. Fat doesn't quiet your hunger. Consequently, people go right on eating the stuff, and put more and more weight on their bodies.

When we examine the effects of these two foods, we get a very different picture from the one that's commonly publicized today. We find that the calories from olive oil are easily converted to body fat and, meanwhile, fail to satisfy your hunger drive—all of which makes dipping your bread in olive oil a much more serious assault on your appearance than, say, sprinkling sugar on your cereal in the morning.

I am not advocating that you eat lots of sugar, especially since it is often found in high-fat foods, but this illustration demonstrates how easy it is to have misunderstandings that ultimately cause us to gain weight. And as I said, this is only one of many false beliefs that make it virtually impossible for you to lose weight and keep it off. By discarding these beliefs and adopting the McDougall Program for Maximum Weight Loss, you'll find that losing weight is not the impossible dream you may have thought it was. In fact, it's actually pretty easy.

The McDougall Program:
For Good Looks and Life

The McDougall Program for Maximum Weight Loss offers you a scientifically sound plan that does not leave you hungry and weak. Because your meals are composed of whole, natural foods, they are nutritionally balanced. The program works because it is based on the latest scientific and medical evidence about nutrition, metabolism, and the hunger drive. It also happens to be an example of the kind of diet that has kept billions of people trim, strong, and healthy for millions of years. Incidentally, that's another fringe benefit of the McDougall Program: While you are losing weight and becoming ever more attractive, your health will improve.

The McDougall Program for Maximum Weight Loss is a no-nonsense program, but the rewards are great. If you choose to follow this diet faithfully, you will undergo a physical and psychological transformation. You should expect to lose between six and fifteen pounds of weight per month, especially if you start out needing substantial weight loss, say thirty pounds or more. (Weight loss slows as you approach trim body weight.) Meanwhile, you will experience greater physical vitality, mental clarity, and self-esteem.

In my previous books, *The McDougall Plan* and *The McDougall Program: 12 Days to Dynamic Health*, I urged people to adopt a starch-centered diet, coupled with moderate exercise, as the basis of a lifelong health program. (You should refer to these books for further information about nutrition and health.) That diet is composed primarily of whole grains and grain products, a wide variety of legumes, vegetables, and fruits. Hundreds of scientific studies have shown that this diet is effective in the prevention and treatment of the most prevalent degenerative diseases caused by the rich American diet. When followed faithfully, the program also results in substantial and permanent weight loss for the vast majority of overweight people.

However, there are many who need a little extra help. I am talking particularly about people with highly efficient metabolisms, many women, people who do not like to exercise regularly, chronic dieters, and those who have trouble getting motivated and sticking to a diet and exercise program. In fact, this group may comprise half of the dieting population. These people need a program that focuses specifically on overcoming the obstacles to weight loss. Consequently, I developed the McDougall Program for Maximum Weight Loss, designed for those who have a single overriding priority: to get rid of unattractive excess weight quickly and keep it off permanently. They want to look great. In the process, they will happily discover that excellent health is a side benefit.

Like the original McDougall Program, the McDougall Program for Maximum Weight Loss allows you to eat as much food as you want. You will still lose weight. Gradually, you will see that your personal appearance is improved through healthier food and lifestyle choices.

The major difference between the original McDougall Program and the McDougall Program for Maximum Weight Loss is that the original diet allows a certain amount of flour products and vegetable foods that are richer in calories. (Chapter 6 contains more information on the differences between the programs, and how you can adopt the original McDougall diet after you've lost all the weight you want to lose, and have kept it off.)

This book provides all the information you need to begin and maintain the McDougall Program for Maximum Weight Loss. It explains the scientific rationale for the starch-based diet, and shows how such a diet cures overweight. Those who have been faithful followers of the McDougall philosophy over the past decade (or more) will gain new tools to help them achieve more control over their appearance. They will find more than 100 new and delicious recipes selected for their weight-reducing benefits.

The weight-loss program is safe and healthy, and can be followed for the rest of your life. (If you are on medication or seriously ill, consult your health care practitioner before changing your diet. Frequently medications must be reduced or discontinued.) However, when you reach the weight that is ideal for you, you can switch to the original program if you wish. It will allow most of you to maintain your weight loss permanently.

The McDougall Program for Maximum Weight Loss works because, like the original program, it is based on the way the body works. When you know the scientific and medical rationale behind the program, you will realize that there are no other options. If you want to lose weight, this is what you must do. And doing it will be easier because it will make sense. One caveat: If you are now seriously ill, it is best to follow the diet under a medical doctor's supervision.

Nobody Can Get Rid of All That Fat

The prime causes of overweight and illness for most Americans are twofold: a rich, fat-laden diet and a sedentary lifestyle. These two factors alone place an overwhelming burden on the human body. Even a highly conditioned athlete may not be able to burn all the calories that enter the system with fatty foods.

In 1990, I was appearing on a talk show in Minneapolis to promote my book *The McDougall Program: 12 Days to Dynamic Health*. Also appearing on the show was world champion track and field athlete Carl Lewis, who, as you probably know, set the world record in the 100-meter dash (9.86 seconds) and won multiple gold medals in the 1988 Olympics. He would do it again at the Barcelona games in '92. While we were waiting to go on the show, Carl explained to me that he was having trouble controlling his weight. It was affecting his running performance. Now, if you saw the '88 or '92 Olympics, you know that Carl Lewis is one of the greatest and best-conditioned athletes of modern times. Yet he was having trouble controlling his weight! Later, in an interview with *Runner's World* magazine (August 1992), he recalled his dilemma. "I had a hard time keeping my weight down," Lewis said. "I never ate—I was starving myself to death to keep that thin racing form. . . . Then I bumped into John McDougall in Minneapolis."

In fact, Carl was having the same problem with fat that most Americans have: There are just too many calories packed into fat for the body to burn away efficiently. Ultimately, fatty foods are going to add weight to your body—even if you happen to be a world-class athlete.

I explained this to Carl and gave him a copy of my book, and he started the McDougall diet. Very soon thereafter, he began to feel the benefits of the program, and shared his experience with others, including his teammates on the world-record-setting 4×100-meter relay team. In the interview with *Runner's World*, Carl said, "I encouraged Leroy [Burrell] and Floyd Heard to try it, too, and we all lost weight. But the big thing was I felt a little better with it, and I've stayed with it."

When asked if the McDougall Program had influenced his performance, Lewis said, "I think it had a lot to do with my performance last year. I'm not saying it made me faster, but it helped keep me thinner and lowered my stress level. It allowed me to eat more consistently and still stay thin." In fact, Carl Lewis set the world record for the 100-meter dash, won two gold medals, and had the best long-jump series of his career (29 feet three times) while on the McDougall Program.

Chances are good that you're not working out every day like Carl Lewis. Certainly I am not. Yet, if he couldn't control his weight on his old diet, how can you or I expect to do it?

The answer is that we can't. This is the immovable fact that causes most overweight people to feel out of control, victimized by food, and condemned to a corpulent figure. Perhaps you have had periods of weight loss that, looking back, seem all too temporary, and all too hard-won. These heroic efforts cannot be maintained forever. But if you believe that you are a failure because you cannot lose weight on the standard American diet—or some facsimile of it—you are wrong. The chances of anyone's losing weight on some version of a high-fat diet are remote.

According to a report from the Council on Scientific Affairs of the *Journal of the American Medical Association*, "Despite a multitude of programs designed to treat obesity, success in treatment often is difficult to achieve. If a 'cure' for obesity is defined as reduction to desired weight and maintenance of that weight for five years, it is more likely that a person will be cured of most forms of cancer than obesity."

This is why people are fed up with diets, and why there is a backlash against dieting in America. As long as you are eating fatty foods, you won't be able to lose weight. You may succeed in starving yourself for a while, and indeed, you may even lose weight temporarily, but that weight will come back for most people. And that causes frustration.

Today, 40 percent of Americans are overweight. When children are eliminated from the numbers, we see that nearly two-thirds of all adult Americans exceed the ideal weight for their height; 25 percent are clinically obese. As long as we go on eating an overabundance of fat, Americans will continue to be overweight.

But there is another component of weight loss that has yet to be widely recognized: our need for carbohydrates.

Eating Fat, but Craving Carbohydrates

Unknown to virtually all of us, we crave carbohydrates. Even in childhood, the nutrient our bodies need more than any other is carbohydrate. Adults need approximately 35 times more carbohydrates for energy than we need protein for growth, and 800 times more carbohydrate than fat. For example, adult men need about 20 grams of protein per day to maintain healthy cell replacement and repair; they need about 700 grams of carbohydrates per day to meet energy requirements; and they need about 3 grams of fat.

Carbohydrates are the most efficient forms of energy that we can consume. Foods that are rich in carbohydrates are vegetables, whole grains, and fruit.

Even while you are eating fat and protein, you are craving carbohydrate. If your diet is deficient in carbohydrates, you will have to eat a great deal more food in an attempt to meet your carbohydrate needs. Along with that large intake of food will come huge quantities of dietary fat, as long as you're eating the typical American diet. The net effect is that you'll be overweight, still unsatisfied, and still hungry.

The McDougall Program for Maximum Weight Loss does exactly the opposite of a carbohydrate-deficient diet. It gives you what you need most (carbohydrate), while it minimizes what you need least (fat), causing you to lose weight. Because the carbohydrates come in foods that are whole, such as whole grains and a wide variety of vegetables, the McDougall diet provides both weight loss and health improvement.

This is why you can eat all you want on the McDougall Program; why you will feel fully satisfied and nourished, and, meanwhile, will lose weight.

These are not unsubstantiated claims, but well-documented facts. The benefits of my program have been scientifically demonstrated. A study of 574 people who have attended my live-in program at St. Helena Hospital in Napa Valley, California, shows that in just eleven days overweight men (weighing more than 200 pounds) lose on the average 8.3 pounds—that's almost a pound a day! Overweight women (who weigh more than 150 pounds) lose, on the average, 4.4 pounds in those eleven days. The people who follow the program lose between 6 and 15 pounds a month, until they approach trim body weight. Most important, these results are attained by eating to the full satisfaction of their hunger drive. Everyone is encouraged to return for seconds, and thirds, if they like. They are cautioned not to remain hungry.

Many of the people who adopt my program, either after reading my books or hearing me speak, do so because it represents a "last resort." Most of them are very discouraged by repeated failure with countless prior efforts. They're on bagsful of drugs, and suffer from a multitude of distresses, dysfunctions, and diseases. They've tried every diet known to the paperback book industry; weight-loss clinics; packaged foods programs; doctor-supervised fasts; and all sorts of medication. They've spent thousands of dollars on expert advice, and they're still overweight.

Because of their progressive downhill course, they believe themselves hopelessly ill and forever overweight. But at this low point their lives turn around, because after all else has failed, they are ready for a big change. That's when they come to the McDougall Program for Maximum Weight Loss.

Those of you who believe that yours is the worst case, let me assure you that you have the greatest potential to be a star on the McDougall Program for Maximum Weight Loss. Many of the men and women written about in this book also believed that they were beyond hope of controlling their weight. And then they adopted the McDougall Program and found that it worked for them. The heavier you are right now, the faster you can improve—and you can do it without hunger. Once you decide to correct the cause of your problems, you will begin to recover.

Marcy Ann Roth, age thirty, of Petaluma, California, is living proof of that. Marcy lost fifty-five pounds, at the rate of about ten pounds a month, on the McDougall Program, and continues to experience benefits. She has been with the program for more than two years. Some time ago, she described her experience this way: "I learned of the McDougall Program from a friend at work. The McDougall diet is the healthiest diet. No more eating from the harmful basic four food groups. Eat, eat, eat, and still lose weight; it's incredible, but true. And the results are almost immediate."

As she lost weight, Marcy discovered other benefits as well. "My cholesterol went from 188 to 131. Also, through the diet and exercise, my body is more toned. I have had to buy a whole new wardrobe."

Marcy had had bad experiences with many diets. "I've tried Weight Watchers, but didn't maintain my weight loss. The disadvantages to this program were: (a) being hungry, (b) eating unhealthy food, (c) having to weigh and measure portions and then keep track of it all. I felt okay on Weight Watchers, just hungry, and when I stopped, then the weight came back."

A Simple Set of Rules

My program is simple to understand and highly effective. I lay out the program in extensive detail in Chapter 6. In Chapter 15, I provide a comprehensive list of packaged and processed foods that can be included in the program. But let me summarize the program here. The foods you should eat include the following:

- All whole grains and whole-grain cereals, such as brown rice, corn, oatmeal, barley, millet, and wheat berries; many packaged grain cereals, puffed grains, and other healthful cereals.

- Squashes, such as acorn, butternut, buttercup, pumpkin, and zucchini.
- Root vegetables, such as potatoes, sweet potatoes, and yams.
- Legumes, such as peas, split peas, black-eyed peas, string beans, and such beans as chick-peas, lentils, and adzuki, navy, pinto, and black beans.
- Green and yellow vegetables, such as collard greens, broccoli, kale, mustard greens, cabbage, various types of lettuce, and watercress; celery, cauliflower, carrots, asparagus, and tomato.
- Fruit, such as apples, bananas, berries, grapefruit, oranges, peaches, and pears. (Limited to two servings per day.)
- For most people, simple sugars, salt, and spices used sparingly at the table rather than in cooking.

These and other foods on the diet make it one of the most interesting food programs on the planet. Once you learn how to use spices, herbs, and various cooking methods, you cannot help feeling nourished and satisfied.

While you are enjoying the above foods, avoid the following:

- All red meat, including beef, pork, and lamb. All are rich in fat, cholesterol, and other harmful constituents.
- All poultry and fish. Poultry has about the same amount of cholesterol as red meat, while fish varies, depending on the type. Some fish are higher in cholesterol than red meat, others lower.
- All dairy products, including milk, yogurt, and cheese. All are loaded with fat and cholesterol. Low-fat dairy products are not recommended because of potential health hazards, including allergies, childhood diabetes, arthritis, and lactose intolerance.
- All oil, including olive, safflower, peanut, and corn oil. Oil is simply a liquid form of fat.
- All eggs. Eggs are abundant in fat and cholesterol.
- Nuts, seeds, avocados, olives, and soybean products (including tofu, soy cheese, and soy milk). Soybean products

are high in fat, unless they have been specially processed (low-fat varieties are also not recommended).
- All dried fruit and fruit juices.
- All flour products, such as breads, bagels, and pretzels. The less a food is processed the better it is for weight loss. Flour products are composed of fragments of grain, or relatively small particles, which increase absorption and slow weight loss.

As you can see, the diet is made up of unprocessed high-carbohydrate foods. Fat is cut to an absolute minimum.

Because the McDougall Program for Maximum Weight Loss has clear boundaries, it is uncomplicated and easy to follow. Meanwhile, you can eat as much as you want and always feel full. Since fat is only 3 to 5 percent of your total daily calorie intake (there is some fat in starches, vegetables, and fruits), almost no fat is left over to be moved to your body fat stores.

Given just a week or two, you will fully adapt to this new way of eating. The first few days require some effort. People must learn the preferred foods, where to find them, and how to prepare them. Within a week, however, they adjust to this new way of eating and find they really don't need meat and fat to enjoy eating. Then the program becomes effortless.

Feasts Become Special Again

The McDougall Program is for daily consumption. It is, essentially, the same diet we humans have been eating for millennia. It is the diet we evolved on, and the diet that is still consumed in traditional cultures and by most of the world.

Our ancestors feasted during celebrations. We ate, drank, and made merry on holidays, in thanksgiving, and on other joyous occasions.

Modern American life is a historical anomaly. Today, virtually every one of us eats as only the few opulent aristocrats once did. The effects of this rich diet on those aristocrats is well documented in medical records and the arts. Paintings of the plump royalty, dressed in their fine robes and dresses, and literary descriptions of decadence and illness attest to the effects of the overindulgence and physical softness of their lives. Let me be clear—I am not making a moral judgment of anyone; I am simply stating a scientific and medical fact: A lifestyle of inactivity and a diet rich in fat and low in carbohydrates destroys human health. We have not been designed by evolution to eat such a diet.

Yet there is a place for rich foods, when and if they are reintroduced into your diet. That place is reserved for festive occasions. If we are to regain our health, turkey must once again be for Thanksgiving, ham for Christmas, eggs for Easter, candy for Halloween and Valentine's Day, cake and ice cream for birthdays. For the average American, every breakfast is Easter, every dinner is Thanksgiving and Christmas; most evenings offer traditional birthday-party foods, such as cake or ice cream or both. If you were to back up and see our lifestyle within the context of the world, or within the context of history, you would see two things: (1) Our eating habits are very different from those of our ancestors, and from those of most of the world today; and (2) these eating habits are the cause of our epidemic of obesity and degenerative disease. The current diet is simply too rich for our metabolism. It is really a matter of balance, of making our daily eating simple and healthful and reserving our feasting for celebrations once again.

It's important that you understand the scientific and medical rationale behind healthful food choices and the McDougall Program. Therefore, I have dedicated the next five chapters to describing the mechanisms by which weight is gained and lost. I've described the essential nature of your hunger drive, your metabolism, and your nutritional needs. In Chapter 6, I offer a complete description of the McDougall diet. In Chapter 9, I describe a safe and effective exercise program that you can stay with easily; and in subsequent chapters I address particular problems (such as why women lose weight more slowly than men). I also discuss how to adapt quickly to the program; how you can maintain the program and still go out to eat in restaurants; and what to shop for in a supermarket. Finally, in Chapters 15 and 16, I present menu plans, cooking techniques, and more than 100 recipes.

So let's begin our transformation, starting with one of the areas that stimulates the most guilt and confusion for people struggling with weight: the body's hunger drive.

CHAPTER 2

The Power of Hunger

Controlling hunger is one of the great difficulties everyone faces when attempting to lose weight. Yet hunger control is the cornerstone of most weight-loss programs. The standard axiom of weight-loss programs is that if you give in to your hunger, you will gain weight. That leaves you with only two choices: Either you mount a Herculean effort to control your natural desire for food, or you take some form of medication or go on a ketosis-producing diet (like the Atkins or Optifast programs) to suppress your hunger pangs. As most people know, these methods usually fail.

What everyone who wants to lose weight must first realize is that the hunger drive was not meant to be ignored or suppressed. It was designed by nature to be powerful, sometimes overwhelmingly so, in order to keep you alive. Therefore, the longer you go without food, the stronger the hunger drive becomes.

For a learning experience, stop eating for forty-eight hours. (Don't attempt this if you are ill or on medication.) The first twelve hours are fairly comfortable. After that you will think increasingly about food. By the time you have been without food for twenty-four hours, you will have discovered a sure way to eliminate all your other daily troubles. You will no longer worry about money, family feuds, or nuclear war. You will have only one thing on your mind—*food!* By the second day without food you will be filling your stomach with gallons of water, desperate for even a temporary feeling of fullness.

If you persist in refusing to eat, your physical discomfort will extend beyond hunger pangs to fatigue, cold, and nausea. These symptoms will grow ever more acute, until you will be unable to distract yourself from your misery.

Without such a strong drive to eat, you might forgo food for play, work, or some other activity. The result would be malnourishment and possibly death by starvation. The unrelenting strength of your hunger drive is necessary for your personal survival—and for the survival of the human race.

Graphic examples of just how strong hunger truly is are scattered throughout history. Hunger has driven people to great acts of courage and ghastly acts of barbarism. But as a general rule, it's safe to say that the hungrier you are, the more out of control you become. You really cannot do very much with your life until you have eaten.

There have probably been times when you have succeeded in controlling this "monkey on your back"—the insatiable desire to eat. Group therapy like Weight Watchers, Jenny Craig, and Nutri-System programs may have helped you sustain your willpower to withstand the pain of hunger a little longer. But, like most dieters, you probably gave up eventually and ate. Once you did, you regained the weight you had lost, and then some.

Hunger Triggers Survival Mechanisms

Regaining weight may have caused you much disappointment and guilt. Many people become angry at themselves and feel like failures. They do not realize that the battle against hunger was never meant to be won. Your own body turns against you in that battle. When you go hungry for a prolonged period, your body reacts as it would to starvation. Studies have shown that the body has a number of survival mechanisms that food deprivation sets in motion. One is a tendency to overeat when food becomes available again, in order to get ready for the next period of food shortage.

After World Wars I and II, victims of starvation found it difficult to control their appetites. Often they would consume 4,000 to 5,000 calories per day, many of them becoming obese. There are reports of prisoners, castaways, and lost explorers who overate, sometimes to the point of death, when food was made available to them after a period of forced semistarvation.

Thus, when dieters stop dieting, they often overeat and regain more weight than they were carrying before they started fasting. Obviously, this can be frustrating, especially given the effort people make to lose the weight in the first place.

People who are starving may also experience improved efficiency of their intestines, which become better at absorbing nutrients after a period of starvation. Thus, when they start eating again, they gain weight more quickly than they did before they began to diet.

Another of the body's survival mechanisms in response to insufficient food is to lower its metabolic rate. With complete starvation, the average weight loss is almost six pounds a week. At this rate, death could be expected in about twenty-one days for a man of average size. However, voluntary starvation in otherwise healthy young men of normal weight can usually be sustained for a little more than sixty days. The survival time is tripled because the metabolic rate drops during periods of food scarcity.

Lowered metabolism means that dieters burn fewer calories both at rest and when they exercise. (See Chapter 9 for more on exercise.) In other words, these survival mechanisms mean that the body works against you when you are dieting. Your intention is to lose weight as quickly and as efficiently as possible; you believe that if you put yourself through a semistarvation routine, weight loss will be easier. But it doesn't work out that way. It's true that you lose weight, but because your metabolism slows and calories are conserved, weight loss requires more effort and more willpower.

Moreover, these survival mechanisms are cumulative. The more you diet, the more efficient your body becomes at using food. Thus, weight loss is slower on the second diet than the first. And each time you begin a new diet, you will have a harder time losing weight, because your body has been trained to survive during periods of starvation. In short, the more you diet, the harder it becomes to lose weight.

It Isn't Just Fat You're Losing, Either

Repeated dieting and weight gain, or the yo-yo syndrome, is not only ineffective but actually deleterious to health because of the kinds of changes produced in body composition. With weight loss during periods of semistarvation, otherwise known as dieting, you lose considerable muscle mass along with fat, especially if you don't exercise while you diet. But after you give up the diet, the weight you regain is primarily fat. The net effect of dieting is that your body consists of more fat and less muscle, at the same weight!

Muscle, which is very active tissue, consumes many more calories than fat tissue. Even while you are resting, healthy muscle burns calories. Fat, on the other hand, is mostly stored calories. Consequently, when you replace muscle with fat, you're actually taking away the very tissues that would help you lose weight in the future. This makes it more likely that you will stay fatter as you convert muscle into fat.

Meanwhile, you blame your appetite for the excessive desire to eat, and you blame yourself for your pitiful lack of will-power. These feelings are reinforced by a chorus of "expert" voices saying, "To lose weight you must cut down," and "Calories are the only thing that count." Overweight people declare, "The reason I'm fat is I overeat. I can't control my appetite!"

Trying to Fool Mother Nature

Faced with this unrelenting hunger drive, people respond in one of five ways:

1. They give up and eat. This naturally results in weight gain, especially on the standard American diet. (You'll see why this happens in greater detail in Chapter 4.)

2. They deny hunger—for a while. A variety of methods are used to deny hunger, but all of them boil down to simple willpower. And as I have been saying, hunger eventually wins out.

3. They take hunger-suppressing pills. Medications are used to deal with illness. People who take diet pills must believe their hunger drive is somehow impaired or unhealthy, and therefore in need of a drug to put it right. These pills result in little weight loss and lots of side effects. Among the most common are nervousness, anxiety, restlessness, irritability, insomnia, dizziness, stomach problems, and dry mouth.

4. They make themselves sick. Temporary illness can be brought about by diets severely deficient in carbohydrates. Without sufficient carbohydrates the body burns fat, producing appetite-suppressing ketones as byproducts. Several years ago these diets relied on carbohydrate-deficient meats and dairy products. These days we have the convenience of "instant sickness" provided by packages and cans of high-protein, low-carbohydrate powders. The results are often dramatic, but the benefits are only temporary (à la Oprah Winfrey). One of the ways they work is by serving as a diuretic, forcing the body to eliminate water from tissues. Eventually, these diets may contribute to disorders of the heart, kidneys, or liver. Because these diets are so rich in protein, they also contribute to the demineralization of bones and can lead to osteoporosis. They can also cause fatigue, poor circulation, loss of appetite, nausea, and irregular heartbeat.

5. They undergo surgery. The seriously obese submit to a variety of surgeries on their intestinal tracts in an attempt to compensate for their hunger. Some surgeries cause greater fullness with less food by effectively shrinking the size of the stomach; staples are placed in the stomach to create a small pouch, or bypasses are performed around the stomach. Other surgeries isolate a portion of the small intestine out of the normal flow of food, causing malabsorption of the foods consumed. These drastic attempts

to "cure" overeating have severe side effects and often are failures.

Whenever you try to manipulate the hunger drive, you are surrendering to one compelling yet erroneous belief: that your need for food is wrong. You believe that nature designed you incorrectly. You therefore believe that your hunger drive must be changed or corrected.

My question is this: Is such a thing possible? Can our biological need for food be out of alignment with our need for health and for stability in our weight? Let's take a closer look.

Understanding Your Human Needs

We are endowed by design with certain instincts and drives that keep us alive and help determine our success in life. These life-sustaining forces can be ranked by how essential they are to life.

Essential Needs

Air: Without air you will survive only three minutes.
Water: Without water you will survive only three days.
Food: Without food you will survive three weeks to three months.

Nonessential Needs

Sex	Family
Money	Occupational success
Love	Community status

The nonessential needs, such as those for sex and occupational success, often rule our lives, but the fact is, we can live without them. On the other hand, we must breathe, eat, and drink to stay alive.

How well has the need to breathe been designed? Do you know people who "overbreathe"? Do you count the number of breaths you take every minute to be sure you get enough air? Or do you rely on the breathing drive? How would you feel if

I told you that there is a shortage of air in your community and that to do your part to conserve, I would like you to take fourteen breaths a minute rather than the eighteen you normally take? It would require enormous concentration and discipline to control your breath continually.

How about thirst? Do you trust your thirst drive? While gardening on a hot summer day, do you say to yourself, "I'm thirsty, but I've already had my six glasses of water, so I can't have any more?" Or do you trust your thirst drive to govern how much you need to drink? How many people do you know who "overdrink" water?

Obviously your drives for air and water were designed correctly and can be trusted. Why is it that so many people "overeat" and must count every morsel that passes their lips lest they become fat and sick? Was the hunger drive designed incorrectly, and therefore not to be trusted? Or are we confusing the hunger drive with something else? The problem is not hunger, any more than it is thirst or the need to breathe. The problem is *what* we eat, not our desire to be satisfied.

Food Offers Choice

Food is unique among our basic survival needs because, unlike our needs to breathe and drink, food offers us choices. The only gaseous mixture you can breathe to stay alive is air, which contains oxygen, just as water is the only liquid you can drink to sustain your life. However, there are hundreds of food choices, everything from antelope sandwiches to zucchini stir-fry. The selections you make among these foods are the primary determinants of your health and your appearance. Therefore, food choices require a combination of instinct (hunger) and the higher faculties of human understanding. We must distinguish what is healthful from what is harmful.

Though poisons have always been with us, the degree of discernment required today is greater than at any other period in human experience. Anthropologists tell us that the earliest human communities, formed some 35,000 years ago, depended on wild grains, vegetables, and berries as their staple foods. For most of human history, we have derived the vast majority of our food from agriculture, meaning cultivated grains, vegetables, beans, and fruit. Animal foods, such as beef, poultry, eggs, and dairy products, were in shorter supply. These special foods were reserved for ceremonial and celebratory feasting. (The idea that these foods are special carried over into the 1950s, 1960s, and 1970s, causing us to see steak as a status symbol.) In traditional societies, nature imposed limits on food availability. Such limits supported health and stabilized weight.

But the United States and much of the Western world have created an agricultural system that provides us with a nearly unlimited supply of beef, pork, poultry, and milk products. Modern technology has also given us refrigeration, chemical preservatives, and a transportation system that can bring the fruits of our agriculture to the far corners of our country and our world. Together, these developments provide us with food choices that were previously unknown in human history.

Now more than ever we must make conscious food choices in order to satisfy our hunger and maintain our health. That requires a certain amount of education and self-understanding. That understanding begins when we throw off the erroneous belief that hunger is the enemy.

Hunger Is Not Your Problem

Your hunger drive is designed correctly. It is intended to keep you alive on this planet, in this body, for as long as humanly possible. In other words, hunger is your friend. It is essential to life and therefore good.

If you are to achieve ideal weight and health, you must change the kinds of foods you use to satisfy your hunger.

This was the experience of Gary Digman of Guerneville, California, a forty-seven-year-old musician and teacher. Like many others, Gary was referred to the McDougall Program by a friend. He had been suffering from overweight and high blood pressure, which eventually convinced him to give the diet a try in March 1990. He is five feet, eleven inches tall and weighed 257 pounds. Since beginning the program, he has lost 60 pounds and has undergone a personal transformation. Gary said: "My skin tone is better; I've got fewer pimples, and my hair is less greasy. Before I started the plan, my doctor wanted to put me on blood pressure medication, but I refused and went on the plan. My blood pressure went from 160/100 to 120/80, with no pills. My cholesterol level is 116. I have fewer colds, and they are much less severe when I do get them. I have more energy, and feel more alert. I certainly have less constipation or diarrhea, and no heartburn or indigestion."

Gary had had lots of experience with other diets. He listed them and their effects on him as follows:

"(1) Fasting—no permanent weight loss. (2) Avoiding salt and red meat—no weight loss. (3) Using low-fat and no-fat dairy products—no success. (4) Low-carbohydrate diet—a disaster. (5) Jogging and tennis—small weight loss, but could not maintain this difficult regimen."

Today, his exercise habits are simple: "I go for a walk for about an hour every day."

Gary summarized his experience on the McDougall diet this way: "The real advantages of the program are simply: It works. No hunger, no loss of energy, no self-denial."

Kathy Clendenen of Healdsburg, California, forty-one years old, had also struggled with an endless list of weight-loss programs, none of which kept her weight off permanently. As she said, "I have spent the last thirty years of my life on diets. Usually my pattern was to restrict my eating to 500 to 800 calories per day, eating such things as spinach and eggs and massive amounts of lettuce. I would lose the desired weight, often thirty to forty pounds, only to put it back on in a few months when I went off the diet. The 'on-off' approach of all my diets was one of my downfalls. When I was on the diet, I felt cheated and resentful. Then I'd make up for it by eating uncontrollably when I went off the diet."

Kathy heard about the McDougall Program from a friend. In three months, she lost thirty pounds and reduced her dress size from 16 to 12. She has been on the program for more than three years. Today, she weighs 130 pounds (she is five feet, seven inches tall).

"The McDougall Program has allowed me a wide choice of foods to eat in an unlimited manner," Kathy said. "It is an 'I can' diet, consisting of great foods, rather than an 'I don't' diet—full of restrictions. Since the diet maintains my weight,

I'm able to take a goodie once in a while. It is also a diet that makes sense—following the patterns of people worldwide for generations."

Kathy walks or uses her NordicTrack for an hour a day three or four days per week.

Besides weight loss, she counts enhanced self-esteem among her benefits. "Because of the weight loss, my self-image has improved, and that translates to many physical benefits. My energy level has increased, and generally my feeling of capability has improved, as I've taken control of my eating patterns. Constipation is something that I've dealt with all my life. This diet has greatly improved that condition as well as that of my menstrual periods."

You *can* control your weight, and do it permanently. But you cannot do it by controlling hunger. Nor can you achieve ideal weight through gimmicky potions, powders, or unbalanced food plans.

In order to lose weight and support your health, you must (1) satisfy your hunger by eating all you need, and (2) eat foods that will help you lose weight and encourage health as you eat. Anything less brings temporary results at best, setting you up for failure and disappointment.

When properly chosen, food will no longer be your enemy. When you follow the McDougall Program for Maximum Weight Loss, you will eat all you want and meanwhile become thinner and healthier.

The foods that give you control over your weight are various starches, with the addition of fruits and vegetables. You must replace your daily fare of meats, dairy products, and desserts with potatoes, corn, rice, beans, squashes, green and yellow vegetables, and fruits. In nutritional terms, this means that all removable fats and oils in your diet must be replaced with carbohydrate. Your hunger drive is satisfied by carbohydrates, not by fat, because carbohydrates are the basic fuel of cellular metabolism. Carbohydrates maintain the body and provide energy.

This is the other secret of hunger: Your body wants carbohydrates more than any other component of your food. And it will urge you to eat and eat and eat until it gets an adequate supply of them.

As you will see in the next chapter, when your body has had sufficient carbohydrates, the hunger drive turns off. Moreover, a meal plan composed of foods high in carbohydrates is four times less concentrated in calories than the typical American diet. Even if you happen to eat more carbohydrate calories than you need, they are burned off as heat or stored invisibly as glycogen (chains of sugars stored in the muscles and liver for later use) rather than as fat. On the other hand, any excess fat you eat is almost effortlessly stored as body fat. High-carbohydrate food also increases your energy and endurance for physical activity, allowing you to burn more calories.

Rich foods must become special again, reserved for festive occasions. Once you have achieved your desired weight on the McDougall Program for Maximum Weight Loss, you can celebrate with a feast. Pick a holiday some months from now, and use it as a target date to achieve your weight goal. In the meantime, follow the McDougall Plan for Maximum Weight Loss. Then, when your holiday rolls around, you'll have something very personal to celebrate. But be forewarned: Once your body gets accustomed to eating well and feeling good again, you may experience a common reaction to harmful foods—indigestion or diarrhea, or what I refer to as McDougall's revenge.

CHAPTER 3

Carbohydrates:
The Secret of Satisfaction

If you and I went for a walk at an elevation of 10,000 feet in the beautiful Sierra Nevadas, our breathing would change dramatically from the way we are used to breathing at sea level. As we got higher into the Sierras, we would experience oxygen deprivation. We would be getting less oxygen per breath than what we are used to getting, and consequently we might have to breathe more quickly and deeply to meet our oxygen needs. As our breaths became deeper and more rapid, we might appear to be compulsive "overbreathers." I could turn to you and say, "Slow down your breathing. You're breathing too much." But what good would that do? You'd be breathing only as rapidly as was necessary to get adequate amounts of oxygen. One way we could cure your "compulsive overbreathing" would simply be to return to sea level, where each breath would bring in more oxygen. Then you wouldn't have to breathe as much to get what you needed. You'd be cured of overbreathing. How wonderful!

Curing people of overeating employs the same principle. Carbohydrates are to hunger what oxygen is to the need to breathe and water is to thirst. Your body craves carbohydrates because they are the body's primary fuel. Of the three primary calorie-providing nutrients in the food supply—carbohydrates, protein, fat—carbohydrates are the most fundamental and cleanest-burning fuel the body can obtain. As you will see shortly, your body is designed to consume and metabolize carbohydrates. And the cells in your body are calling out constantly for an adequate supply of carbohydrates. Consequently, satisfaction of hunger depends on your getting enough of them from your diet. As long as your diet is deficient in carbohydrates, you will be hungry. Your stomach may be temporarily full, but you will still be yearning for what your body needs. To use the metaphor of breathing at high altitudes again, you must breathe more—that is, eat more—to get what your body is craving. Let's take a closer look.

The Need for Carbohydrates

Our digestive tract, beginning with the mouth, tongue, teeth, and saliva and proceeding to the stomach (via the esophagus), the small intestine (where nutrients are absorbed), and the large intestine (from which waste is eliminated), is designed both to enjoy and to efficiently use carbohydrates. I say enjoy because even the tongue and taste buds were designed to select for carbohydrates. We are rewarded for eating the foods our bodies need. At the tip of the tongue are the "sweet" taste buds, indicating that the sweet taste is the one we want to experience first and foremost. This biologic sweet tooth—or "sweet buds"—provides for gustatory pleasures that make us happy to select the foods we need most. It's nature's way of ensuring that we do what we're supposed to do to keep the body going. More on the top of your tongue, toward the front, are the taste buds for salty flavor. Farther back, along the sides of the tongue, are the taste buds for sour flavor, and in the very rear, the taste buds for bitter flavor.

Anthropologists tell us that ancient humans learned early that sweet taste indicated nutritious foods, while bitterness often suggested poisons. If a food didn't taste sweet right at the tip of the tongue, it was discarded, and the body was protected.

Sweet tastes are found in complex and simple carbohydrates. The foods that are rich in complex carbohydrates are starches, such as grains, beans, potatoes, and vegetables. Simple carbohydrates, which are highly concentrated, are found in many fruits and various sweeteners, including honey, barley malt, maple syrup, and refined white sugar.

The design of our teeth is consistent with this pattern of carbohydrate selection. Our front teeth are shaped with cutting edges to break off pieces of starches, vegetables, and fruits, which are then ground by the flat molar teeth at the sides and back of the mouth.

While being chewed, food is also mixed with saliva. The saliva contains the digestive enzyme alpha amylase, whose sole function is to break down complex carbohydrates into simple ones that can be easily absorbed through the digestive tract.

The reason the body selects for carbohydrates above all other nutrients is that our greatest need is for fuel. Even in childhood, the body needs much greater quantities of fuel for cellular metabolism than protein for growth. Not only do carbohydrates provide the greatest abundance of fuel, but they also are the cleanest-burning fuel available to the body. Carbohydrates are composed of carbon, hydrogen, and oxygen, and their main by-products when metabolized, carbon dioxide and water, are both easily eliminated from the body. Protein, which can be used as fuel, requires much greater effort to convert to energy, and its by-product, nitrogen, converts to ammonia and urea, both of which can be harmful, especially in higher quantities.

But the mouth and its many characteristics are just the beginning. Your entire digestive system is designed to process large amounts of carbohydrate efficiently. The first part of the small intestine contains digestive juices made by the pancreas that are also rich in carbohydrate-digesting amylases. The intestine is long and convoluted, allowing for the slow and complete process of digesting carbohydrates.

When examined for what it handles best, the anatomy and physiology of the human intestine are revealed as the perfect factory for the digestion and assimilation of foods high in carbohydrates. It is the entire digestive process that gives us a feeling of being fully satisfied.

Hunger Is More Than Being Filled

Hunger is more than a mere need for bulk. If bulk were all we needed, we could satisfy ourselves on tire rubber. But hunger is a marvelously complex yearning to satisfy a complete range of nutritional needs. Hunger will not subside until we are nutritionally satisfied, and that satisfaction will not occur until we have consumed sufficient carbohydrates.

Although filling the stomach may provide some initial relief, hunger will not go away until food enters the small intestine, where the food's components, particularly its carbohydrates, are absorbed into the blood and distributed to cells. Because of the paramount role played by carbohydrates in human nutrition, it follows that their ingestion satisfies the appetite as no other component of the food can. If you fail to consume sufficient amounts, you will continue to be hungry (for carbohydrates). The result will be that you will likely overeat from all food groups—which will include lots of calories from fat and protein—in your efforts to consume sufficient carbohydrates.

No wonder so many traditional cultures have made grains, tubers, and legumes the center of their diets. Hunter-gatherers consumed tubers as their starch; agrarian communities turned to seed crops. In Europe, wheat and corn are the main seed crops; in Asia and Africa, people consume rice and millet. Starchy roots, such as yams, cassava (a starchy root, also called manioc), and potatoes are common in tropical regions.

The Eating Contests

As I mentioned in Chapter 1, I run a twelve-day live-in health program at St. Helena Hospital in Napa Valley, California. At each session, we get a lot of overweight people; inevitably, one or two will weigh in excess of 300 pounds. They describe a fairly common dilemma: They're able to consume tablefuls of food at a single meal, yet they're still hungry. After hearing their tales of gluttony, I challenge them in a voice loud enough for everyone at the dinner table to hear: "I'll bet I can eat more food than you can!" These mighty eaters gladly accept my challenge.

On the first day, they will take two or three large platefuls of food at each meal from our cafeteria-style service. (I will keep up with or surpass their portions. Predictably, they lose the eating contest, because I am used to eating these foods at this early time and they're not.) By the third day they will declare that one medium plate of food is all they can eat. I tell them, "You're not getting your money's worth. Eat more!" They respond, "I'm full!" I smile, having known they would be satisfied by the high-carbohydrate diet. These good sports have helped make a point. "You see," I say to them. "You can be satisfied by your food after all."

At last, they are satisfied and full. After so many years of stuffing themselves with the wrong foods and depriving themselves of what they really yearn for, they find themselves satisfied—finally—by carbohydrates.

Starving for Carbohydrates in America

The rich American diet is made up primarily of carbohydrate-deficient foods. Meat, poultry, and fish have no carbohydrate. Nor are there any carbohydrates in lard, butter, olive oil, corn oil, or any other vegetable oil. Cheese has only 2 percent of its calories as carbohydrate, cottage cheese only 8 percent. Obviously, these foods will not satisfy your carbohydrate needs, and consequently they will not satisfy your appetite. On a carbohydrate-deficient diet your body keeps saying to you, "When are you going to feed me? Maybe the next plateful will contain what I need?"

When you consume a diet that's deficient in carbohydrates, your eating usually stops when you're stuffed. At that point, your stomach is distended by that high-protein, high-fat food, and you're in pain. Meanwhile, you're still longing for the satisfaction that can come only from carbohydrate-rich foods.

Addicted to Ice Cream?

Many people tell me they are addicted to cake, ice cream, and candy. They talk about their overwhelming cravings for sugar-laden foods. On a carbohydrate-deficient diet sugar is often the only significant source of carbohydrate available. Because of its pure concentration of carbohydrate, sugar provides a powerful reward for your deprived taste buds—a jolt of stimulation.

After your breakfast of bacon and eggs—both devoid of carbohydrates—you long for the reward of two tablespoons of sugar in your coffee. A lunch centered around breast of chicken leaves you starved for the sugar in your after-lunch candy bar. That thick, juicy steak for dinner doesn't quite satisfy until it is topped off with cake and ice cream. Without this sugar fix you're bound to feel unsatisfied. Then the satisfaction arrives with a bang. The concentrated sugar in desserts and snacks after a meal of fat and protein is an exhilarating experience, like the first gulp of fresh air after swimming the length of the pool underwater. Cigarette smokers can draw an analogy to the especially satisfying pleasure of that first cigarette in the morning after hours of abstinence. I can understand why some people consider chocolate ice cream and candy an addiction; the ecstasy from eating concentrated sugar after chewing through a dinner of carbohydrate-deficient foods is like a fix to an addict deprived of drugs.

Stop the deprivation and you stop the cravings. When you spend your entire meal consuming carbohydrates, you satisfy your needs and desires with every bite. You are not left longing. A dessert at the end of the meal loses its powerful impact because your hunger has already been satisfied.

The table on the following page shows the carbohydrate content of various foods. You can see how dramatically foods vary in their carbohydrate content.

FOOD	PERCENT CARBOHYDRATE
Almonds	13
Apples	100
Asparagus	77
Avocado	15
Bacon	0
Barley	90
Beef	0
Blackberries	89
Butter	0.2
Carrots	92
Cheddar cheese	2
Chicken	2
Codfish	0
Corn, sweet	94
Eggs	2
Grapes	91
Kidney beans	72
Lobster	1
Margarine	0
Milk (whole, 3.5% fat)	30
Oatmeal	71
Olive oil	0
Peanuts	14
Potatoes	90
Pork	0
Rice	86
Shrimp	0
Sunflower seeds	14
Sweet potatoes	92
Tomatoes	85
Tuna	0
Turkey	0

Fat and Protein Provide Little Satiety

Studies performed on rats in the middle part of this century gave rise to a series of incorrect concepts about human nutritional needs and appetite. Because laboratory animals maintain their energy levels on very different kinds of diets—everything from high-fat to high-carbohydrate diets—scientists were led to believe that fat satisfied human hunger better than carbohydrate.

However, later research demonstrated that human hunger is quite insensitive to fats in the diet. There are no taste buds on the tongue for fat, for example, and no basic drive for fat, except the one learned through many years of repeated experience and the accrual of psychological associations with high-fat foods.

Eighty percent of what we perceive as taste is actually smell. Our faculty for taste is the least acute of our five senses. Thousands of molecules of any substance must dissolve on the tongue before the tongue can perceive a taste from that substance. Smell, on the other hand, is among the most acute of our senses. We can detect an odor by encountering only nine molecules of a substance. When you experience what you call taste, your brain is actually combining information from both your taste buds and your olfactory nerves, which you interpret as taste. Our dependence on smell is revealed every time we have a cold; once the nose becomes stuffed up, we lose the capacity to taste anything, simply because we cannot smell it.

In the Western diet, most of the flavors and smells are tied up in fat-soluble molecules. Consequently, we associate rich flavors with high-fat foods, such as steak, gravy, cheese, and ice cream. Asian diets are precisely the opposite: Most of the flavors and smells in the Japanese and Chinese diets are tied up in water-soluble molecules. The foods that provide such tastes are grains, vegetables, fruits, and water-based sauces. The Asian diets are also highly aromatic, meaning that their range of flavors is complex and satisfying. But the water-based tastes in Asian diets emerge from low-fat foods, and these regimens are therefore much more healthful. The Japanese and Chinese have learned to enjoy, even crave, the very foods that maintain health. So can you.

Taste preferences are not driven by genetics, but by education. You learn to like the foods you currently choose. Mexican children, for example, find hot peppers repugnant when they first encounter them, thanks in part to the presence of a natural irritant called capsaicin. But because adult family members enjoy the peppers, the children develop a taste for them. They learn to like a substance that naturally irritates them.

Food preferences are learned and unlearned. We can expand the list of foods we currently enjoy simply by giving our palates time to appreciate them. Meanwhile, if we avoid certain foods, we soon find ourselves repulsed by the dishes we once thought enjoyable. In other words, food choices are highly changeable. They are based almost entirely on time, experience, education, and associations. This is why people who adopt the McDougall Program for Maximum Weight Loss find themselves, after a short period, enjoying foods they were unaccustomed to. Given a week or so, whole grains and a vast variety of vegetables and fruits begin to taste both delicious and satisfying.

Meanwhile, you're meeting your carbohydrate needs and losing weight at the same time.

Carbohydrates Satisfy Emotional Needs

Carbohydrates have effects on the body that extend beyond physical health to emotional and psychological well-being. In fact, they change brain chemistry to relieve depression and decrease the hunger drive.

Research at the Massachusetts Institute of Technology has demonstrated that carbohydrate consumption increases levels in the brain of a chemical neurotransmitter called serotonin. Serotonin, MIT researchers have found, triggers a sense of well-being, improves the ability to concentrate, and enhances sleep. It also diminishes hunger. By eating carbohydrate-rich foods, we increase the level of serotonin in our brains, and consequently enjoy all these benefits.

Foods rich in protein, such as meat and dairy products, have the opposite effect on brain chemistry: They cause a relative decrease in serotonin levels.

We all use sweet foods to deal with our moods. People who suffer depression in light-deprived environments, or during winter (a condition known as seasonal affective disorder, or SAD), often crave carbohydrate-rich foods to counteract this effect. Many women crave chocolate and other carbohydrate-rich foods just before their menstrual periods to relieve irritability and depression. Obese people intermittently consume excessive amounts of carbohydrate to improve their mood and deal with anxiety. It all works because carbohydrates increase levels in the brain of serotonin, which in turn improves mood.

This is also why people who adopt the McDougall Program find themselves feeling better emotionally after a short while.

The McDougall Program has made believers out of a lot of skeptics. People come to my program from all walks of life— athletes, businesspeople, blue-collar and white-collar workers. Yet they all have a few things in common: They've been following the typical American diet for decades; they're either sick or overweight, or both; they have tried other programs and failed; and they are ready to try the McDougall Program as a last-ditch effort.

That was the experience of Mike Ferreira, forty-three years old, from Santa Rosa, California, who had tried a lot of diets before hearing me on a local radio talk show. Mike said, "I started doing the diet gradually, but changed over completely because of arthritic knee and back pains. In four months I went from 215 to 174 pounds and then stabilized at about 185. I have now been eating a starch-based diet for two years. This program works! I would advise people to try it for just two to three weeks. If you're honest with yourself about your intake, that should convince you. Be fully informed about what you're eating. There are a lot of misleading traps, such as food labeling."

Besides weight loss, Mike has seen other benefits. "Most of the back pain is now gone, and my arthritic knee pain is completely gone. I used to take ibuprofen for them, but don't need that now."

Joey Hadfield of Wilsonville, Oregon, was sixty-six when she adopted the McDougall Program. After she heard me on *The Larry King Show*, she bought one of my books and adopted the diet. In six months, she dropped forty pounds and three dress sizes and took five inches off her waist. Two years later, the forty pounds are still history. Joey said she is about 80 percent faithful to the diet, having about four feast days a month. Yet she stays trim, and still she eats more and feels much better than ever before.

One of the great things about the McDougall Program, Joey said, is that she is full after each meal and does not feel the need to cheat or snack. If at any time she feels a craving for something, she eats.

Joey exercises for about forty minutes each day on an Airdyne stationary bike. Besides the weight loss, she also reports, "My skin tone is better, my eyes are brighter, and friends tell me I look much younger. I used to always have an upset stomach—that's gone now. I was always constipated and now I'm regular every day. I'm also much less nervous."

Like many others who have come to the McDougall Program for Maximum Weight Loss, Joey has a long history of diets. She said she lost twenty-five pounds at a national weight-loss center. However, after several months she developed an ulcer; her doctor told her that the center's program "was the worst way to diet with my history. On another program I lost twenty pounds, and this seemed to be better on the ulcer. With both plans I was always thinking about *food!* After stopping these programs, I not only gained back the weight, but I gained more. I was constantly constipated too."

Lisa Caldera of Windsor, California, was only twenty-six when she started the McDougall Program for Maximum Weight Loss, which helped her lose six pounds. "I saw Dr. McDougall on *People Are Talking.* I tried the program for two weeks and realized how much better I felt. I used to have the worst Jekyll-and-Hyde personality, due to PMS. Every minor little thing would cause major stress in my life. I would get so depressed I would cry at the drop of a pin." All these conditions have changed for the better, Lisa said. "My nasal discomfort, due to hay fever, has also improved. I don't get sick unless I push myself too hard at work. The increase in energy was also a big improvement. I can work circles around the old me, who was always tired."

Permanent Control Through Satisfaction

The solution to controlling your hunger drive is to give your body the carbohydrates it longs for. You might as well begin satisfying your needs right now. When I say eat, I mean it.

Because of your past experience, many of you will find my insistence that you stuff yourself with starches, vegetables, and fruits difficult to accept. But the sooner you get started, the sooner you will be on the road to permanent control of your health and appearance.

CHAPTER 4

The Second Secret:

The Fat You Eat Is the Fat You Wear

All of us have been trained to think that weight loss involves counting calories and limiting our intake of them. The formula is so simple and so compelling that few people look more deeply at the issue of weight loss. They accept the axiom as an ultimate truth.

Now I come along and tell you it's all a hoax. Counting calories and fasting are like putting a mouse on a treadmill; the mouse has the experience of making a great effort, but in truth it's not going anywhere. If the mouse wants to make any progress, it has to get down off the treadmill and start walking on land.

That's what I am telling you. The standard approach to weight loss is really a treadmill that will keep you in the same circle of experience: Initially, you are inspired and hopeful about a new diet; you fast, suffer hunger, and count calories; you enjoy short-term weight loss; the hunger takes its toll and you break your fast and eat. Never having understood the true mechanisms for weight loss, you naturally go back to your old way of eating, which will cause you to regain the lost weight and then some. After all that time and effort, you're back where you started, just like the mouse. Even worse, you feel like a failure. What you do not realize is that fasting and calorie-counting are a treadmill. They're not going to get you anywhere.

The reason current methods fail is that they do not address the importance of satisfying hunger, our need for carbohydrates, and the hidden source of guaranteed weight gain in everyone's diet: fat.

So let's turn now to the second secret of weight loss in the McDougall Program for Maximum Weight Loss: the role of fat in the diet.

Fats are calorically dense foods. In other words, they are concentrated sources of calories—in fact, the most concentrated forms of calories available. A gram of fat provides approximately nine calories, while a gram of pure carbohydrate or a gram of pure protein provides only four calories. That's one of the reasons I say that a high-carbohydrate diet will not provide you with as many calories as your fat-rich American diet will.

Fat is called a high-energy food because it provides lots of calories per gram, meaning that every fatty meal we eat provides lots of potential energy, or lots of potential for obesity.

Before we go any further, let me point out that a calorie is not a mysterious entity. It's just a measurement of potential energy in a given fuel. A single calorie is one unit of potential energy. Most Americans need between 1,800 and 2,500 calories each day for their bodies to run efficiently. Lumberjacks and professional athletes, of course, need more, but since most of us work in offices or at other sedentary jobs, our needs are relatively similar.

Just because fat provides lots of potential energy doesn't mean that fatty foods will give you lots of energy. Actually, fat is easier to store than it is to burn as fuel. Your body will burn all the available carbohydrates before it burns significant amounts of fat. Thus, even though fat is considered a high-energy food, it is really a high-storage food, because in real life your body tends to store much of the fat you consume in your diet.

Many Kinds of Fattening Fats

No doubt you have read or heard about various kinds of fats: saturated, polyunsaturated, and even monounsaturated. These words indicate the type of chemical structure associated with each fat.

Fat molecules are comprised of carbon, oxygen, and hydrogen atoms. The more hydrogen atoms there are in each molecule, the more saturated the fat is. Think of a fat molecule as a living room with a certain amount of space. Saturated fats are rooms that are filled to capacity with furniture; you couldn't squeeze another end table in there. Monounsaturated fats have some room still available for a chair or two, and polyunsaturated fats have even more room for, say, a sofa, a love seat, and a few odds and ends.

Like the room that's stuffed with furniture, the more saturated a fat is, the denser it is. Saturated fats are so dense that they tend to be solid at room temperature. A stick of butter is a saturated fat. Most saturated fats are found in animals, and so they are often called animal fats.

Vegetable fats are usually monounsaturated or polyunsaturated fats. Each of these has fewer hydrogen atoms stuck between their carbon atoms. ("Mono" indicates one unfilled bond; "poly" indicates many bonds where hydrogen could be added.)

While saturated fats tend to be solid at room temperature, mono- and polyunsaturated fats are liquid at room temperature; that is, they are oils. Oils are liquid fats. In nature there are no free fats; they are all mixed up with other components of foods. Oils are freed from their original food source by various processing methods, which may be as simple as grinding peanuts and skimming the oil from the surface.

A few vegetable fats are predominantly saturated. These include coconut, palm oil, and cocoa butter.

You've seen corn oil or soybean oil labels that read "partially hydrogenated." This means that hydrogen atoms have been stuffed into a mono- or polyunsaturated fat, which makes the corn oil or soybean oil solid. Once it's solid at room temperature, it can be used as an imitation butter, or margarine, or shortening for frying or baking.

A saturated fat is not only dense, but packed with calories, or potential energy. Mono- and polyunsaturated fats are slightly less dense, but because they are fats, they too are packed with calories.

The fattiest foods in the plant kingdom are avocados, nuts, seeds, olives, and soybeans. Most plant foods are low in fat, while most animal foods tend to be high in fat, especially those foods Americans commonly consume. The greatest sources of fat for most Americans are meats, poultry, fish, dairy products, processed packaged foods, and a variety of vegetable oils.

Regardless of the kinds of fats you eat, all are easily stored.

It's Easy to Make a Pound of Body Fat

Your body will always make the most efficient use of the raw materials provided at the dinner table. As you saw in Chapter 3, the body's favorite fuel for daily activity is carbo-hydrates. Proteins in the diet are used for building and rebuild-ing tissues. Everyone's diet, no matter how unhealthful it is, is made up of a combination of carbohydrates, proteins, and fats. Since the body prefers carbohydrates as fuel, it will use them first. It will also burn some fats. However, since most of us live fairly sedentary lives, and at the same time eat lots of fat, much of the fat we eat will be transferred to fat cells for storage. The preferred destination of the fats in your diet is your adipose (fat) tissue, which lies just below the surface of the skin and surrounds your internal organs.

Still, fat is used for more than just energy. A small amount of fat—less than 4 percent of your total daily calorie intake—is used for synthesis of new cells, hormones, and other body parts. Another 3 percent of calories is burned in the transfer of fat from the dinner plate to the adipose tissue. That leaves 93 percent of the fat consumed. Guess where that goes? You guessed right: It's stored in your tissues, to be used when en-ergy needs are not being met by carbohydrates.

All this transportation is accomplished so efficiently that the original chemical structure of the fat is maintained. If samples of your fatty tissues were extracted with a needle for analysis in the laboratory, the results would reveal the kinds of fats you usually ate. If you ate large amounts of olive oil, the analysis would show predominantly monounsaturated fats, the same as the original olive oil. If you ate margarine and shortening, the test would show predominantly a "trans" form of polyunsaturated fats. A diet high in fish fat would cause your fat cells to be filled with omega-3 oils. If animal fat was the largest part of your diet, your body fat would be mostly saturated.

Because their dietary fats come primarily from animals, Americans have higher levels of saturated fats and lower levels of unsaturated fats than people living in Japan, where the diet is lower in animal fat and higher in vegetable fat.

Since more than 90 percent of the fat you eat is being stored, it means you need to consume only 3,765 calories of fat to make one pound of body fat. Under these circumstances, you need to eat only a few meals of fatty foods to add a pound of fat to your abdomen, hips, or thighs.

Consider that in one week you could make a pound of body fat if you were to use daily:

- three ounces of cheddar cheese on each of your two lunch-time sandwiches, or
- four and a half tablespoons of olive oil in your evening-meal pasta sauces, or
- three tablespoons of blue-cheese salad dressing on your lunch and your dinner salad, or
- one eight-ounce sirloin steak for dinner,
- or one bowl of ice cream for a nighttime snack.

In a month you could make a pound of body fat by daily use of:

- four strips of bacon for breakfast, or
- four pats of butter or margarine spread on your breakfast toast, or
- one generous knifeful of mayonnaise spread on your lunchtime sandwich, or
- two knifefuls of peanut butter on your sandwich, or
- one tablespoon of safflower oil to grease your pan for a stir-fry, or

- one piece of coffee cake at your morning or afternoon break.

Each pound of stored fat represents 3,500 calories. That's more than a full day's energy needs. Twenty-five pounds of fat will meet your energy requirements for about fifty days. The adipose mass of an ordinary person is between twenty and forty-five pounds. This volume of fat is similar to the size of all the muscles, the skeleton, or the skin. The adipose tissue can increase 1,000 times in size, yet lean tissue can shrink and enlarge by only two to three times.

All of that fat is really potential energy that may never be needed if you maintain your current diet and level of exercise. However, even exercise cannot save you if you continue to add pounds of fat to your body by consuming a high-fat diet. In other words, it is very hard to get rid of fat unless you change the composition of your diet from high-fat to high-carbohydrate.

The expression "from my lips to my hips" is an accurate description of the ease with which fat from your fork and spoon is transformed into body fat. (We'll see how this efficient process makes it easier for many overweight people to gain weight.)

Importance of Fats, Proteins, and Carbohydrates

Fat is more than a backup energy supply. It is used by the body to metabolize certain vitamins (A, D, E, and K), to insulate and support organs, and to maintain cell membranes.

The human body is quite capable of synthesizing most kinds of fat. However, certain fats which cannot be synthesized are required for growth, maintenance, and proper function of many physiological processes. These "essential fats" must be obtained from the diet. The most important essential fat is linoleic acid. When you don't get enough linoleic acid, you can suffer from dry, scaly skin and other symptoms; a deficiency of linoleic acid in infants causes inadequate weight gain.

Your need for essential fat is less than 2 percent of the calories in your diet—probably as low as .55 percent of calories. It is practically impossible to cause a deficiency in essential fat in adults. Even if you stopped eating fat entirely—a virtual impossibility, since all natural foods contain some fat—there is still a large supply of essential fat stored in your adipose tissues. That supply is sufficient to meet the needs for those fats in adults.

Interestingly, essential fats are synthesized only by plants, not by animals. Therefore, a diet composed of plant foods—even those very low in fat—provides an abundance of essential fat to meet human needs.

Cellulite Is Nothing Special

Many people believe that cellulite—the fat that often collects on the hips and legs—is especially resistant to dieting. Cellulite occurs mostly in women, and in some obese men on the abdomen. As everyone knows, cellulite is particularly unattractive, having a "cottage cheese" look. This dimpling of the skin is created by the combination of protein fibers and fat tissue; the former binds, the latter expands, creating the appearance of an unevenly stuffed mattress. The only realistic solution to cellulite is to unstuff the mattress, which means eliminating the underlying fat and thus taking the tension off the fibers. This will cause the skin to become smooth.

With weight loss, cellulite begins to disappear. (I discuss fat reserves on women's hips and cellulite more fully in Chapter 7.)

But What About Protein?

Americans always wonder about protein. Somewhere back in the 1950s, people became convinced that the most important nutrient in the food supply was protein, and whenever you suggest a change in diet, somebody always asks the same question: "Will I get enough protein?" As I explained in my first book, *The McDougall Plan*, you get plenty of protein on the Mc-

Dougall Program, because vegetable foods provide it. But let's look a little more closely at our protein requirements.

The Fate of Protein

Digestion of protein begins in the stomach, where acids and enzymes begin to break it down into smaller components called amino acids. Some of the protein is immediately used to build muscle, skin, hormones, and other tissues. Most of us use very little protein each day. Exceptions are growing children, body-builders, and people recovering from injury. Studies have shown that an active, healthy adult man uses less than 20 grams of protein a day.

Americans consume an average of 160 grams of protein daily, or about eight times what we need. Little, if any, is ever used as energy. Nor is protein converted into carbohydrate, unless there is none available in the diet. Likewise, protein is not converted to fat. There is no place for storage of any of the excess 140 grams of protein the average American consumes each day. The truth is, you've got to get rid of it.

All that excess protein is processed and eliminated by the liver and kidneys. In the process, this leftover protein over-works these organs. As a consequence, they become enlarged and the kidneys slowly deteriorate over a lifetime. The loss of kidney tissue is insignificant for most people because of their reserve capacity. Normal function is maintained with as little as one-quarter of the kidneys. However, someone who has lost kidney tissue from an accident, diabetes, atherosclerosis, an infection, or another cause can suffer life-threatening damage to the kidneys from a diet that contains as much excess protein as the typical American diet.

Excess protein also causes changes in kidney metabolism. Minerals are also lost from the kidneys in large amounts when they are called on to eliminate the excess protein, particularly animal protein. Among the most important minerals lost is calcium from bones, which can lead to osteoporosis and kidney stones. Most of that damaging protein comes from animal sources, such as red meat, poultry, dairy products, eggs, and fish.

Only in the most desperate situations, such as severe illness or prolonged starvation, will the body use the protein in the tissues as fuel. People desperate to lose weight will often starve to lose. The body happily burns fat. But unfortunately, proteins from muscle and other important tissues also are consumed to survive. This is like burning your own house, or at the very least like burning your best oak furniture in your fireplace, rather than ordinary wood, to survive the cold.

Converting Carbohydrate to Fat— A Rare Event

If protein isn't stored as fat, the question arises: Is excess carbohydrate stored as fat? Here again, the answer is no. The body always uses the most efficient means of processing the components of the foods we eat. Converting carbohydrates to fat is metabolically very costly. Therefore, almost all of the excess carbohydrates we eat are simply burned and released as heat through the skin and lungs, rather than being converted into fat.

The standard American diet provides about 250 grams (1,000 calories) of carbohydrate a day. Most of it is used immediately to provide for daily energy needs. If more carbohydrate is available than can be used, the initial excess is stored in the liver, kidney, and muscles in long chains of reserve fuel (or sugar) called glycogen.

Carbohydrate storage contributes very little to your weight. Your total stored reserves of carbohydrate—your glycogen— amounts to 2,000 to 4,000 calories, which is equal to 500 to 1,000 grams, or one to two pounds of glycogen. This does not have much effect on your scale. Nor on your figure, since the carbohydrates are stored invisibly in the liver and muscles.

On a starch-based diet, in which 85 percent of calories consumed are derived from carbohydrate, a normally active man would have to consume 5,000 calories a day before his body would resort to converting the excess into significant amounts of fat. This would mean eating more than twenty-five cups of cooked rice or thirty-three large potatoes daily. Very few people could sustain such a feat for more than a few days.

The bottom line is that carbohydrates do not add weight to your body. Dietary fat leads to body fat. In other words, the fat you eat is the fat you wear.

Avoiding fat, on the other hand, causes the fat you're now wearing to be burned away quickly.

John and Roberta Ray, of Butte, Montana, forty-nine and forty-four years old, respectively, lost fifty pounds each by following the McDougall Program—and they did it without thinking about fat or calories or controlling their hunger drive.

"My sister in Vancouver, Washington, heard Dr. McDougall on TV and bought the book, and then told us about it," Roberta said. "Immediately after reading the book we started the program. John's cholesterol dropped 100 points. I used to have one or two severe colds every year. I have no colds with this way of eating, and more pep and energy." Roberta got eleven members of her family on the McDougall Program; collectively they have lost 250 pounds.

Cal Kimes, of Santa Rosa, California, forty-eight years old, lost sixty pounds and experienced many other health benefits after he adopted the McDougall Program.

"The program was recommended to me by a business partner and my cardiologist," Cal said. "I was generally feeling unhealthy and decided to start it. I weighed in at 280; I now weigh 220 and went down two suit sizes. It took me four months to accomplish this. I am never hungry. I want to lose another ten to fifteen pounds, and will do it by just staying on the diet. My cholesterol dropped from 267 to 173. My slight diabetes is now in the safe range. I stopped taking my blood pressure medicine."

As John, Roberta, Cal, and many others have found, eliminating fat from your diet is the quickest and surest way to lose weight. It's also one of the fastest ways to improve other aspects of your health.

CHAPTER 5

Calorie Dilution and Insulin Control:

The Third and Fourth Secrets of Permanent and Effortless Weight Control

Regardless of what we may eat, we're all looking for the same thing: satisfaction from our food. For those interested in losing weight or improving their health, the question is this: How do I achieve maximum satisfaction from my diet, lose weight, and strengthen my health at the same time? Many people believe that this is asking too much. We are trained to think that satisfaction is bad when it comes to weight loss or health improvement. But if you follow the McDougall Program for Maximum Weight Loss for a week or so, you will learn that you can be fully satisfied—even happy with your diet—while you lose weight and improve your health. That's what this diet does. But short of feeding you myself, I must show you how such a thing is possible. So in this chapter you'll discover just how satisfaction is really achieved.

Satisfaction: Where It Starts

As we all know, food satisfaction begins with taste. But the need to taste food is more than psychological. When scientists introduce food directly into the stomach by feeding a person through a tube, they find that hunger satisfaction is actually delayed. Obviously, the sooner you are satisfied, the sooner you stop eating. And if satisfaction is delayed, you'll keep on eating until you are sated, which, from the standpoint of weight loss, is not good. In other words, it's important that you enjoy your food, from both a psychological and a physiological standpoint.

To do that, you must begin by chewing it thoroughly. Digestion of carbohydrates begins in the mouth. Your saliva contains the enzyme ptyalin, which breaks down carbohydrates and prepares them for digestion. The more these carbohydrates are broken down in your mouth, the sweeter your food becomes. Saliva dissolves your food, so that it becomes more accessible to your taste buds. Together, the ptyalin and saliva enhance your ability to taste and enjoy your food, which makes it possible to feel sated by less food.

The same mouthful of food can provide very different degrees of satisfaction. One mouthful that is not fully chewed will provide less satisfaction than an equal portion of the same food that is well chewed. You can prove this to yourself with the following experiment. For a day or two, keep track of how much you eat for breakfast, lunch, and dinner on the McDougall Program for Maximum Weight Loss. Then, over the following few days, eat the same foods, but this time chew every mouthful thirty-five to fifty times. You'll notice that each mouthful will become more satisfying than your previous meals. You'll also notice that you are fully satisfied—even stuffed—on far less food than you were the previous few days. Chewing changes the level of satisfaction you experience from your food. It enhances your ability to enjoy a food's flavor. Therefore, the more you chew, the more you enjoy and the sooner you are satisfied. Chewing is another secret of efficient weight loss.

Filling the Stomach Satisfies Hunger

After taste, the second requirement for satisfaction is the feeling of fullness. None of us wants to be hungry, no matter how determined we are to lose weight. The feeling of fullness alone plays a major role in our food satisfaction, because once the stomach is full our need for food diminishes.

Filling the stomach causes distention of the organ, which in turn triggers a message to the brain that food has been eaten. Once you've eaten to capacity, your stomach will signal you that it's "full," to which your brain says, "No more food." Bulk alone has long been known to alleviate hunger.

But as we all know, your stomach can be filled—and satisfied—by a wide variety of foods, everything from hamburgers and other high-fat foods to grains, squashes, and other foods rich in complex carbohydrates. Each type of food will have a different impact on your weight, because each food contains very different amounts of calories.

Food: Combinations of Nutrients

All foods are made of various combinations of five major ingredients—fats, proteins, carbohydrates, fiber, and water—and several minor components, including vitamins, minerals, and contaminants. Animal foods contain cholesterol. The relative amounts of fat, protein, carbohydrates, fiber, and water in your chosen foods will determine how many calories wind up in your stomach.

Obviously, some foods are far more calorie-dense than others. Here are the calories found in a gram of each of the five main food ingredients:

Fats	9
Proteins	4
Carbohydrates	4
Fiber	0
Water	0

These numbers become even more revealing when we look at specific foods. Consider the number of calories you would have eaten if you filled your quart-sized stomach with about two pounds (1,000 grams) of the following:

FOOD	CALORIES
Beef	2,920
Broccoli	273
Brussels sprouts	385
Cauliflower	242
Cheddar cheese	4,028
Corn	1,085
Garbanzo beans	1,188
Orange	464
Pumpkin	336
Potatoes	860
Rice	1,190

Of the five major components of food, only three—protein, carbohydrate, and fat—can be sources of calories. The fourth component, water, provides no calories, but is essential for most of the body's processes. The last, dietary fiber, provides no calories either, because it is not absorbed into the body. It passes through the digestive tract; but as you will see, it enhances digestion and improves satisfaction immensely.

Since water and dietary fiber contain no calories, foods rich in these constituents have fewer calories, while those that are low in both likely have more. Starches, vegetables, and fruits are high in fiber and water

Fiber: For Satisfaction and Health

Dietary fiber is found only in plant foods. There is no fiber in beef, chicken, fish, eggs, or milk. Fiber is not like the bristles of a brush. Rather, it is made of long branching microscopic chains of simple sugars that are connected by linkages that resist digestion.

Fiber is a wondrous food constituent. As it passes through the digestive tract, it helps to eliminate cancer-causing substances as waste. But it also performs other important functions. For example, fiber binds with fat and cholesterol and eliminates them in the feces. This, of course, causes a decrease in calorie absorption—eliminating some of the fat that would otherwise become part of our tissues—and lowers blood cholesterol levels. Fiber also increases the activity of the bowel (a process called peristalsis), thus improving elimination of waste and unused calories.

Additionally, fiber binds with water and thus increases the volume of the food in your stomach and intestines, which brings satisfaction sooner and with fewer calories. Fiber also slows digestion enough to prolong the feelings of fullness.

Studies have shown that high-fiber diets prolong eating time, enhance satiety, and improve the body's capacity to use energy. High-fiber foods tend to be rich in complex carbohydrates, a source of long-lasting energy. But fibrous foods also increase the sensitivity and efficiency of insulin, the hormone that makes sugar available to your cells. (More about insulin shortly.) When insulin is made more sensitive and efficient, less insulin is needed to bring blood sugar to cells. As you will see, keeping insulin levels low is important in weight loss.

The Role of Insulin in Weight Reduction

Insulin is a hormone produced by the pancreas; its job is to regulate the amount of fuel in your bloodstream. It controls your levels of glucose (or blood sugar, the body's main fuel) by helping to transport glucose from the blood to your cells.

Eating causes your pancreas to produce more insulin, and it does so in great quantities—usually between five and seven times the amount that was present before eating.

Having more insulin in your blood means that your body will burn more blood sugar. That's why you sometimes get that quick energy buzz after you eat a piece of fruit or some sugar. But you also burn these quantities of energy quickly, which will rapidly lower your supply of blood sugar. Once the supply drops, your body signals your brain that more fuel is needed; that stimulates your appetite, which encourages you to eat. Thus, the higher your insulin level, the more energy is burned, and the sooner your appetite rises.

In this way, elevated insulin leads to increased appetite and increased food consumption. Insulin is a key to appetite. Therefore, in order to control appetite and lose weight, you must keep your insulin low.

Insulin Governs How Much Fat You Burn

Not only does insulin increase appetite and lower blood sugar, but it also governs how much fat you burn.

If you were to fast, your insulin would fall, which would allow your fat reserves to leave your fat cells to provide energy to your body (a process called lipolysis). However, when you eat, insulin simultaneously causes an increase in fat production (a process called lipogenesis) and fat storage, while it inhibits the breakdown and release of fat from your adipose tissue. In other words, you store more fat and you burn less stored fat.

In short, insulin promotes obesity by:

1. Increasing appetite.

2. Increasing fat deposition.

3. Inhibiting fat release.

Factors That Elevate Insulin

In general, high-carbohydrate, high-fiber, low-fat foods make insulin work more efficiently and reduce the amount of insulin needed by the body and produced by the pancreas. On the other hand, high-fat foods dramatically increase insulin production. Refined foods, like white bread, white pasta, and white rice move rapidly into the blood and cause a surge of insulin production too. Sugar produces an even more exaggerated insulin response.

One reason refined foods elevate insulin is the absence of fiber. As you saw earlier, fiber improves insulin efficiency, meaning that less is necessary to do the job.

Insulin's relationship to gaining weight is well illustrated by diabetics, who are usually overweight, especially those with type II, or adult-onset, diabetes. People with diabetes often take pills that increase the pancreas's output of insulin. As a result, diabetics often become obese and have a difficult time with weight reduction.

The following list summarizes the factors that elevate insulin and contribute to weight gain:

Obesity
High-fat foods
Sugar
Refined foods
Infrequent meals
Physical inactivity
Diabetic pills (oral hypoglycemic agents)
Insulin injections

A Vicious Circle—Obesity and Raised Levels of Insulin

It has long been known that most obese people have elevated levels of insulin in their blood. Obese people are caught in a vicious circle: They have a higher insulin level, which promotes hunger, which causes them to eat more, which puts on weight; the more weight they carry, the higher their insulin level, the more easily fat is stored, the more they gain weight.

But the whole process is reversed by weight loss, which lowers insulin, lowers appetite, and leads to greater weight loss. The McDougall Program for Maximum Weight Loss is the most effective way of breaking out of this vicious circle.

Keeping Your Insulin Low

High-complex-carbohydrate foods, especially those high in fiber and low in fat, move slowly through the intestinal tract. The fiber causes the carbohydrate to move into the bloodstream in a slow, even fashion. In this way, it reduces the amount of insulin needed to deal with the incoming sugar. Also, physical activity uses up blood sugar and reduces the need for more insulin.

Diabetics on insulin must keep their sugar under reasonable control, but they should also avoid taking too much insulin, which will stimulate the appetite and encourage accumulation of fat. Diabetic pills (oral hypoglycemia agents) are hazardous to health and cause weight gain. I never give them to patients. A customary prescription for diabetics is to lose weight in order to get their diabetes under better control and prevent complications such as heart disease, stroke, and cancer. Therefore, it seems like a contradiction to give medication that makes the patient fatter, which, in turn, makes the diabetes worse.

The Proof Is in the Weight Loss

I have provided you with lots of scientific information, and it can be effective as a tool for your intellect. But never forget this one truth: The proof is in how you look and feel. As you follow this way of eating, you will feel better and look better. Ask George H. Mills, fifty-two years old, who lost ninety pounds.

George, who lives in Santa Rosa, California, was introduced to the program by his dentist, who gave him a copy of *The McDougall Program*. In the first six months of the program, George's waist went from sixty to fifty-two inches and his weight from 390 to 300 pounds. "My normal color has returned, and I no longer take insulin, Prozac, and Lomotil," George said. "I am always full. I eat three times as much food as ever before. I have more energy." And George continues to lose weight.

George is lax in his exercise program: "I do light walking about three times a week."

His previous attempts at weight control have been many: "I tried urine of pregnant women [a weight-loss shot]: lost 40 pounds, gained 60. I tried Weight Watchers: lost 100, gained 120. Hypnosis—nothing! Acupuncture—nothing! I even had a major heart attack and lost 120 pounds in the hospital, and gained back 150 pounds. I tried a liquid diet: lost 50 pounds, gained 70 pounds."

Unlike George's other experiences, the McDougall Program has worked. "I have already recommended the program to ten other people," he said. "They see my great loss and it wins them over."

For forty-eight-year-old Jollena Tylor of Camarillo, California, the McDougall Program for Maximum Weight Loss has meant both a youthful figure and the skin of a much younger woman.

"A friend who attended Dr. McDougall's lecture in Vancouver, British Columbia, told my husband and me about the program. We read *The McDougall Plan*, and attended the health center. I have lost thirty-eight pounds. I went from a dress size of 14 to 16 to an 8 to 10. I have never been hungry. I eat more now than I did. I used to skip breakfast. Now, I eat bigger, starchier lunches, about twice as much. I look younger—friends say ten years younger. My skin is clearer and my large pores have normalized. The muscles in my legs have firmed. Cellulite is nearly gone from my thighs and bottom. My face, chin, and neck muscles have better tone, and have certainly slimmed over. Now I have a freedom which comes from overcoming the restrictions of being too heavy. I can bend, stoop, get up and down without awkwardness. No more shoulder pain, either." She has been on the program since May 1991.

CHAPTER 6

The Maximum-Weight-Loss Program:

The Diet

The McDougall Program for Maximum Weight Loss is based on the original McDougall Program, with certain modifications to make weight loss faster and easier. The program consists of two parts: a dietary regimen and an exercise plan. To get the best results, you should follow both parts of the program. However, the dietary plan alone should cause you to lose between six and fifteen pounds per month. I say that with two qualifiers: The first is that I assume you need to lose a substantial amount of weight, say thirty pounds or more. The diet alone causes most people to lose weight until they've reached a weight close to their ideal, at which time their bodies naturally achieve an equilibrium between the calories they take in and those they expend. The second qualifier is this: You must follow the diet faithfully to lose weight. Halfway measures do not work well, because they usually involve cheating with high-fat, low-fiber foods, which, as I have shown, contribute to weight gain.

As long as you need to lose weight and you follow the program carefully, you will lose weight effortlessly. The diet will do this by itself, but if you have trouble losing the last ten to twenty pounds, you should increase your exercise and follow the "rapid-weight-loss" track of the program, which includes more green and yellow vegetables (see below).

The Maximum-Weight-Loss Eating Plan

The eating plan of the McDougall Program for Maximum Weight Loss is a new way of eating. The diet is composed mostly of starches. The main categories of these starches are:

- Whole grains, such as brown rice, barley, oatmeal, wheat, and millet.
- Potatoes, sweet potatoes, and yams.
- Squashes, such as acorn, butternut, buttercup, summer squash, and pumpkin.
- Legumes (beans, peas, and lentils)
- Yellow and green vegetables—such as carrots and collard greens. These are important additions.
- Fruit. The program limits fruit to two servings a day.

These foods are scientifically proven to provide optimal, balanced nutrition, and therefore are ideal for all human beings, no matter what their weight. However, because of their high carbohydrate content and low fat content, they are ideal weight-loss foods.

The maximum-weight-loss eating plan is easy to follow. As long as you stay within the food guidelines presented here, you can eat whatever you want, and as much as you want. No complicated calculations are involved.

1. Eliminate All Animal Foods

This means no meat, poultry, fish, seafood, eggs, milk, butter, cheese, yogurt, or sour cream. As I have explained, many of these foods are extremely high in fat. Most contain no carbohydrates. The carbohydrate in milk, lactose, is not digestible by most people in the world, and in many people the protein in milk contributes to bone loss and a variety of allergic disorders. Animal foods contain no fiber, which satisfies hunger, regulates blood sugar and insulin, and maintains healthy bowel function.

Besides these problems, animal foods contain cholesterol

and have serious vitamin and mineral deficiencies. Animal foods are also dangerously high in protein, which contributes to kidney damage, kidney stones, and osteoporosis.

2. Eliminate All Oils

Remember, oil is pure liquid fat, containing nine calories per gram. That fat will end up in your tissues and contribute to weight gain. It will also significantly raise your chances of contracting a serious illness, including cancer, heart disease, gallbladder disease, and diabetes, to name just a few.

3. Eliminate All High-Fat Plant Foods

High-fat plant foods include nuts, nut butters (such as peanut and almond butter), seeds, seed spreads (tahini), avocados, olives, coconut, and soybean products, including tofu (which is 54 percent fat). These vegetable foods are high in fat, which is effortlessly stored in your adipose tissue. They provide only meager amounts of carbohydrate to satisfy your hunger. Because these foods are not of animal origin, many people are fooled into thinking they are "health foods." For this reason, there are many overweight vegetarians with oily skin and hair.

4. Eliminate All Flour Products

Eat your grains whole. Eliminate breads, bagels, pastas, pretzels, crackers, and corn and wheat tortillas. In general, the less a food is processed, the better for weight loss. Grinding changes two major characteristics of the food: First and most important, grinding a whole grain into flour increases the surface area of the food exposed to the intestinal tract, which increases the amount of nutrition absorbed in the intestines. This also increases the rate at which carbohydrates enter the bloodstream, where they raise insulin and blood sugar. Grinding a whole grain into flour increases absorption of calories and the rise in blood sugar and insulin by three to four times. Second, grinding disrupts the dietary fiber, thereby reducing its ability to slow absorption, lower insulin, regulate blood sugar, satisfy appetite, and enhance elimination.

5. Eat Whole Grains and Potatoes

All whole grains (such as rice, barley, millet, wheat, and oats) and potatoes (including sweet potatoes and yams) fall into the category of starches. They are rich sources of carbohydrate and fiber, which help satisfy hunger, slow digestion and absorption, and reduce insulin secretion by the pancreas.

6. Eat Legumes

Legumes include all beans, peas, and lentils. Legumes have a protein coat and high soluble fiber and carbohydrate content. These factors cause them to be digested and absorbed into the bloodstream slowly. The carbohydrate in legumes requires that they be digested in the last part of the small intestine, the ileum, which signals the stomach to slow the release of food. This contributes to the feeling of fullness you have when you eat beans and other legumes. It also contributes to the feeling of fullness you get from your next meal, which may be four or five hours later.

The same factors that contribute to fullness and slower digestion also keep insulin levels in the blood lower, even when legumes are blended or mashed.

7. Make Green and Yellow Vegetables One-Third to One-Half of Your Meal

Compared with most starchy vegetables, green and yellow vegetables have about one-fourth the calories.

To lower the overall concentration of calories in your meal plan, replace some of the starchy vegetables with green and

Starchy Vegetables

FOOD	CALORIES/GRAM*
Beans	1.3
Corn	1.1
Lentils	1.2
Potato	0.8
Rice	1.1
Sweet potato	1.0
Winter squash	0.4

Green and Yellow Vegetables

Asparagus	0.3
Broccoli	0.3
Cabbage	0.3
Cauliflower	0.3
Eggplant	0.2
Lettuce	0.2
Mushrooms	0.3
Onion	0.3
Tomato	0.2
Zucchini	0.2

* Doctors, dietitians, and scientists compare the calorie concentrations of foods by dividing the number of calories by the weight of the food. This results in a number referred to as the calorie density of the food. For example, the calorie density of a raw potato would be figured by dividing 88 calories by 112 grams, which equals 0.8 calories per gram.

yellow vegetables, but not so much that your meals become unsatisfying.

8. Eat Uncooked Foods

Regular consumption of raw vegetables will cause you to lose weight faster. Carrots, celery, broccoli, cauliflower, zucchini, snow peas, bell peppers, and onions are commonly eaten raw. Eat your two fruits a day uncooked.

Cooking begins the breakdown of complex carbohydrates

into more easily digested, sweet-tasting simple sugars. You may have noticed that grains, vegetables, and fruits taste sweeter after they are cooked. A popular sweet-tasting bread called Essene or Wayfarer's Bread is made sweeter by slowly cooking the sprouted grains at a low temperature. Cooking may also decrease the particle size of many foods. Simpler sugars and smaller particle size increase the speed with which such foods are digested, raising insulin and glucose and thereby slowing weight loss.

9. Restrict Fresh Fruit to No More Than Two Servings a Day, and Avoid Dried Fruit, Fruit Puree, and Fruit Juice

Fruits are relatively low in calories. The following table shows just how low:

FRUIT	CALORIES
Apple	81
Banana	105
Grapefruit	37
Mango	135
Orange	65
Peach	37
Pear	98

The problem with fruit is that it's so tasty you could eat twenty pieces a day, and in the process consume an extra 1,000 to 2,000 calories, which will, of course, slow weight loss. Fruit sugar causes significant increases in blood fats (triglycerides) in some people. These fats are the very ones stored in fat tissues. Fruit also stimulates insulin production, which stuffs these fats into fat cells.

Processing fruit into sauce or juice disrupts and/or removes fiber, increasing the speed of absorption and the amount of carbohydrates absorbed by the bloodstream. Fruit puree, such as applesauce, raises insulin more than whole fruit. Fruit juice causes even greater insulin production.

Dried fruits contain concentrated calories. Purged of its water, dried fruit is less filling than fresh fruit. You would be hard pressed to eat three whole apricots (a total of 153 calories) in the time it takes you to read this page. But you could easily— and quite unconsciously—eat ten dried ones (for a total of 510 calories) in that time.

10. Use Simple Sugar Sparingly

Common simple sugars, such as white sugar, brown sugar, fructose, honey, molasses, maple syrup, and concentrated apple juice, all slow weight loss.

They do this in two ways. First, by providing calories, sugar spares the burning of body fat and slows fat loss. Second, sugar is a strong stimulus for insulin production. Insulin encourages the storage of fat in the fat cells.

Here's how to use sugar on the McDougall Program for Maximum Weight Loss. One teaspoon of sugar contains only sixteen calories of carbohydrate. Eliminating these few calories from your diet will make little or no difference in your weight, but a teaspoon of sugar may determine whether or not you eat your oatmeal. For this reason, the McDougall Program allows small amounts of sugar on the surface of food. But sugar is not allowed in cooking, where mixing with the food covers up the pleasurable taste. Also, foods that contain combinations of sugar and fat are strictly forbidden. And these combinations are more plentiful than you may realize.

In the standard American diet, sugary foods or sweets usually mean cakes, ice cream, doughnuts, and chocolate candies. All of these are actually mixtures of fat and sugar. This combination may be especially fattening because the sugar stimulates production of insulin at the same time that large amounts of fat are entering the bloodstream. The net effect is dramatically increased fat storage. The sugar and fat content of many candies, cookies, and desserts makes up 98 percent of the calories.

Making Healthful Substitutions

Although the guidelines above seem specific, they need some elaboration. The following table lists specific foods to avoid and what to use instead. In addition, the "McDougall-Okayed Packaged and Canned Products" are listed in Chapter 15.

DON'T USE	POSSIBLE SUBSTITUTES
Milk (for cooking)	Rice milk (a drink made from brown rice, water, and a sweetener)
Milk (for drinking)	Water, herbal tea, cereal beverages
Butter	None
Cheese	"Cheese" Sauce (recipe page 219)
Yogurt	None
Sour cream	None
Ice cream	None
Eggs (in cooking)	Ener-G Egg Replacer
Eggs (to eat)	None
Meat, poultry, fish	Starchy vegetables, whole grains, legumes, winter squashes
Mayonnaise	None
Vegetable oils (for pans)	None: use Teflon, Silverstone, Baker's Secret (silicone-coated) pots and pans
Vegetable oils (in recipes)	None; omit oil or replace with water or mashed banana for moisture
White rice	Whole-grain rice or other whole grains
Grain flours	None

Guidelines for Healthy Eating

What you eat is, of course, the key to the program. But how you eat is important too. The following principles are helpful for successful weight loss.

1. Eat Until You're Satisfied

Contrary to popular thinking, the more you eat, the thinner you will become. The important qualifier is that you must eat the foods listed on the McDougall Program for Maximum Weight Loss. When you're full, you are not as strongly tempted to eat foods outside the program. A stomach full of well-prepared high-carbohydrate, low-fat foods effectively curbs your tendency to cheat yourself out of great looks and great health. Meanwhile, you'll appear to be a tower of strength and discipline to those around you—and you'll feel like one.

2. Graze

Eat six or more small meals a day and snack frequently on the recommended foods.

Studies have shown that obese people tend to eat fewer but larger meals than lean people. This research challenges the time-honored belief that we should eat three "proper" meals a day and not snack in between, at least when weight loss is the goal. Eating only one or two times a day conveys a message to the body that food is only intermittently available, and that real scarcity might be right around the corner. Therefore, we are programming ourselves to eat more when food is available to us, which encourages the body to go into survival mode, to slow metabolism, and to efficiently use all calories.

When gorging is your eating pattern, your body uses some of the food immediately, but stores the rest in anticipation of the time when food will not be available. (I discussed the consequences of such survival mechanisms in Chapter 2.) Also, the longer you are deprived of food, the tastier the food seems when you finally eat, the longer your meal lasts, the faster you consume food (especially at the beginning of the meal), and the more you ultimately eat.

Just thinking of food increases the body's metabolism and causes the expenditure of calories, a phenomenon known as cephalic thermogenesis. Thus, the more often you eat, the more often you think of food and the more often you expend energy through cephalic thermogenesis. All these factors point to the fact that you should eat frequently—of the recommended foods—to lose weight more effectively.

3. Allow Time for Digestion

Time is needed for the stomach and intestines to tell the brain that you have eaten and satisfied your nutritional needs. This is especially important on a diet high in carbohydrate, because satisfying hunger is accomplished by meeting your carbohydrate needs rather than by stuffing yourself. If you allow a little time for the foods to pass into the small intestine and the carbohydrates to enter the bloodstream, you will be fully satisfied, and you'll eat less.

As a guideline, eat in the following way:

Fill your plate with a reasonable amount of food. After you have finished that portion, wait about twenty minutes for digestion to start. You will find your hunger drive diminishing quickly. If you're still hungry after twenty minutes, have seconds and again wait. This is a variation on the importance of frequent meals. You move from a gorging pattern to grazing, with greater satisfaction of hunger and less calorie intake.

4. Chew Foods Thoroughly

Satisfaction from our food begins in the mouth. Increased chewing results in greater satisfaction of the appetite. Not surprisingly, high-fiber vegetable foods also require more chewing. In addition, taking time to chew your meals, rather than speed-feeding them, allows the stomach and intestines to communicate to the brain that your nutritional needs have been satisfied and you can stop eating.

5. Restrict Variety

The number of calories consumed has been found to increase with variety. As a food is eaten, its appeal in taste and appearance decrease, but the taste and appearance of other foods remain relatively unchanged. As a result, more is eaten during a meal consisting of a variety of foods than during a meal with just one food, even if that food is a favorite.

In many parts of the world, the bulk of a population's food intake comes from one staple starch food, such as rice in Asia. In these places, obesity is unknown. Simple diets, centered around starches, are still consumed by most of the world's population (China, Japan, Africa), and they are very nutritious. These people do not suffer from the hedonistic appetites of those of us in the West, where a great variety of food is the norm. Here in the West, obesity is commonplace. Consider that the average supermarket contains 15,000 to 20,000 items.

You might be worried that restricting variety could lead to malnutrition. Throughout life we have been brainwashed by marketing messages touting "a well-balanced meal." However, nutritional research clearly shows that a diet based on a single starch with the addition of a fruit or a vegetable provides all the protein, essential fats, vitamins, and minerals required for adults and children. Even extreme examples of diets based on simple starches have been shown to be nutritionally adequate.

Orphaned and abandoned children as young as eight months living in Peru have been raised with normal growth patterns while consuming white potatoes as their sole source of nutrients. Oil was added to their diet to provide extra "empty" calories.

Adults have lived for long periods in excellent health on potatoes and water alone. Oil was again added to the potato diet to provide more calories because of greater-than-desired weight loss from this starchy diet. (When oil, a source of empty calories, is added, the protein, mineral, and vitamin concentration of the potatoes is diluted. Still, all nutritional requirements are met, further attesting to the superior nutrition in simple foods.)

Vitamin and Mineral Supplements for Your Program?

Many of the restricted diet plans you have tried before may have recommended you take vitamins. After all, they reduced the amount of food you consumed and therefore reduced necessary nutrients. The McDougall Program for Maximum Weight Loss encourages you to consume unlimited quantities of nutrient-rich foods—plentiful in proteins, carbohydrates, essential fats, vitamins, and minerals; therefore, supplementation is unnecessary, except for one vitamin made by bacteria (B_{12}). (Grains and legumes do require the addition of foods richer in vitamins A and C, like a fruit or green vegetable, to be completely nutritious. However, root vegetables, like potatoes, are plentiful in both vitamins.)

Eleven of the thirteen known vitamins are made by plants; therefore, a diet of plant foods is especially rich in these vitamins. Vitamin D is really a hormone synthesized in your skin with the help of sunlight. Sufficient sunlight is necessary for good health. The last vitamin, B_{12}, should be taken as a supplement if you are going to follow an all-vegetable diet like the McDougall Program for Maximum Weight Loss for more than three years, or if you are pregnant or nursing. Most people get adequate amounts of B_{12} from bacteria in their intestine and in the environment. To guard against the unlikely possibility of a deficiency, a daily supplement of 5 micrograms of B_{12} is plenty for most people. An alternative is to check blood B_{12} levels yearly; above 150 picograms/milliliter is evidence of sufficient body stores of this vitamin.

Plants contain an abundance of minerals; therefore, mineral deficiency, including calcium and iron deficiency, is never a problem on a starch-based diet. Supplementation of minerals is unnecessary and sometimes unwise. For example, calcium supplements will inhibit the absorption of iron into the body.

Serious Simple Treatment of Obesity

One of the most effective and famous weight-loss diets used over the past fifty years was developed by Walter Kempner at Duke University. Kempner's Rice Diet consists of 400 to 800 calories a day, most of which (90 to 95 percent) comes from rice, fruit, and fruit juice. Later in the program, vegetables are added, along with small amounts of lean poultry or meats. In a review of the weight-loss benefits, 106 massively obese people were shown to have lost an average of 141 pounds in approximately one year. Forty-three of the 106 achieved normal weight. Men lost more weight than women. The authors concluded, "This study demonstrates that massively obese persons can achieve marked weight reduction, even normalization of weight, without hospitalization, surgery, or pharmacological intervention." Yet no nutritional deficiencies have been found; this weight-loss program has a long history of safety.

Dr. Kempner has had extraordinary success using this program to treat a wide variety of diseases, including acute and chronic kidney diseases, enlarged and diseased hearts, diabetes, hypertension, and obesity. Other well-documented improvements in health include a decrease in blood sugar, triglycerides, and uric acid. Improvements in electrocardiogram abnormalities, eye disease (retinopathy), and enlarged hearts have also been reported. Dr. Kempner's pioneering work is a landmark in helping people with a simple starch-based diet.

Nature's Variety on the McDougall Program

The McDougall Program for Maximum Weight Loss offers an incredible variety of vegetable foods. Once you are familiar with these foods, you will not feel deprived or think your diet lacks variety. The vegetable kingdom offers the most healthful source of variety in the food supply.

A Few Further Considerations

These additional ideas for weight loss may have some small value to you.

Fiber supplements may increase weight loss by reducing the proportion of food that is digested, and by lowering blood insulin and blood sugar. Use either soluble fibers, such as guar gum, oat bran, or rice bran; or insoluble fibers, such as wheat bran. The soluble fibers are particularly effective at lowering insulin and blood sugar.

Including salt may stimulate the appetite, increasing calorie intake, and may also accelerate the digestion and absorption of food. The absence of salt makes food less palatable. Thus, cutting down on or avoiding salt may increase weight loss. To increase palatability, you can use a small amount on the surface of the food, where the tongue contacts it, but whenever possible avoid salt in cooking, where it provides less taste. Salt-free seasonings are also helpful. (See Chapter 15 for "McDougall-Okayed and Canned Products List.")

Hot red pepper (capsaicin) may increase the metabolic rate and burn more calories, thus promoting weight loss. Use it judiciously in place of salt. Cayenne pepper and dried red pepper flakes are convenient sources of capsaicin.

Artificial sweeteners may impede weight loss by increasing hunger (by decreasing brain serotonin levels and increasing insulin). Since a little sugar is allowed, there is no need to use saccharin, aspartame, or other artificial sweeteners.

Water may fill the stomach and create a sense of fullness without providing calories; in this regard, it does not contribute to weight gain. However, drinking water may also increase the flow of food out of the stomach, causing quicker return of hunger and faster digestion and possibly increasing the tendency to gain weight. Therefore, drink only when you are thirsty and try to avoid drinking at meals.

Be Faithful to Yourself

The McDougall Program for Maximum Weight Loss works, as long as you follow it faithfully. You can fail yourself. Little lapses can make the difference. Because of the efficient design of the human body, the preferential destination of any fats added to the starch-centered diet will be your hips, thighs, belly, and chin. You may very well be eating better than ever before, but that may not be enough. Or you may not be eating as close to the rules as you have led yourself to believe. As one famous diet pioneer has said, "All dieters are liars." Researchers commonly describe the difference between what people actually eat and what they report as the "eye-mouth gap." The one who loses out by failing to follow the principles of the McDougall Program for Maximum Weight Loss is you. Review the principles regularly and check your daily eating habits against them.

Balancing Your Meal for Weight Loss

You can increase the speed and efficiency of your weight loss by eating more green and yellow vegetables, salads, and side dishes. But these foods must be balanced with the greater satisfaction provided by the more luscious starchy dishes in your meal. Recipes for weight loss are provided in Chapter 16. The only difference in these three modifications of the McDougall Program for Maximum Weight Loss is in the proportion of starch versus vegetable dishes:

Moderate—Two-thirds starch and one-third very-low-calorie salads

Rapid—One-half starch and one-half very-low-calorie salads

Hasty—One-third starch and two-thirds very-low-calorie salads

Look over the recipes for both starchy dishes and low-calorie green and yellow vegetables in Chapter 16. Pick one recipe from each grouping for your meal. After preparing these dishes, serve them in portions that fit your weight-loss approach. You can determine how much you want to eat with an "eyeball" estimate. Weighing is unnecessary. Results do not require such precision. Ideally, the very-low-calorie green and yellow vegetable portion of the meal should be consumed before the starchy portion; this will ensure that the lower-calorie foods are consumed before you are full.

I recommend a moderate approach for everyone who first attempts the McDougall Program for Maximum Weight Loss. Most people will get excellent results and will certainly find the meals tasty and satisfying. The rapid approach will result in even faster and greater weight loss, and can be recommended to anyone who is impatient or is moving too slowly toward his or her goal weight. As the name ·implies, the hasty approach may result in very rapid weight loss, but may not be the wisest approach for permanent weight loss: You may find that satisfaction from the meals may be too low for long-term adherence. However, stoic people who love green and yellow vegetables may find this the best approach, for whatever period they prefer. With this large volume of low-calorie vegetables, everyone—even those who are sedentary, with highly efficient metabolisms—will find weight loss effortless. (Only cheaters will fail to lose weight using this approach.)

Karen Nichols, twenty-nine years old, of Rosebury, Oregon, thought I was a "fanatical vegetarian" when she first heard about me and said she would never have read my books or listened to me speak on her own. However, her sister-in-law, who was very concerned about her health, gave her my books and encouraged her to read them, which Karen did.

Karen had tried plenty of other diets, but she was hungry all the time, a condition she says she couldn't deal with. Yet "counting calories worked pretty well till I stopped doing it. I'd lose weight on 1,000 calories a day, but I was hungry all the time, and got plenty sick of salads. Plus I gained all the weight right back.

"The reason I never started a diet like this," Karen said, "is I never thought that meat and dairy products were bad for me.

'They' told me I needed them since the first grade. How could I know not to eat them?"

Karen was five feet, seven inches tall. She had recently given birth, and during her pregnancy her weight had shot up to 192 pounds. As so often happens, she couldn't get rid of the extra pounds after the baby was born. "I was nursing my baby, so I could not go on any of the usual diets." After reading our books, she decided to try the diet.

During the first six months, she lost forty pounds, and she has kept them off for over two years (since 1991). During her most recent pregnancy, while following the McDougall Program, she only gained 19 pounds. At five feet, seven inches tall she now weighs 140 pounds. She wants to lose about ten pounds more, but has had a hard time staying away from refined sugars, oils, and breads and muffins made with oil. But she is working on it and hopes to find inexpensive, tasty oil-free breads.

"The McDougall Program is not really a diet I'm on, but is simply a major change in the way I eat and feed my family. I will never go back to eating the way I did before. I have no desire to eat those foods anymore. The few times I tried, I got diarrhea and stomach cramps. I haven't tried meat in months because I think it would give me a stomachache as well."

Karen's only exercise is about an hour of walking twice a week. Meanwhile, she has experienced numerous other benefits. Among them is a remarkable change in the condition of her hair, which her husband, Brent, now refers to as "glowing." She also feels much more energy and is much happier. "I've bought all new clothes—the old ones don't fit." She used to take ibuprofen frequently for headaches, which are almost all gone now.

When You Reach Your Desired Weight

The McDougall Program for Maximum Weight Loss is not a gimmicky weight-loss program that you discard for your ruinous eating habits the moment you achieve your weight goal. In order to maintain your weight loss, you must continue to follow the program. Why would you want to return to the rich American diet anyway, when you look and feel so much better now?

Look at the principles of the McDougall Program for Maximum Weight Loss not as a prison but as a set of tools. Once you have maintained your desired weight long enough to appreciate fully the control you have—perhaps six months—then you may want to reintroduce the slightly higher-calorie foods allowed on the original McDougall Program. Most people can do this without noticeable weight gain. If you find moderate use of breads, bagels, pastas, pretzels, crackers, more cooked foods, dried fruits, juices, fruit purees; fewer green and yellow vegetables; and occasional high-fat plant foods undesirable, then head right back to the principles of the McDougall Program for Maximum Weight Loss.

You will figure out how much of these "less-thinning foods" you can tolerate before you start to regain weight. That tolerance will depend on your level of exercise, the number of times you fall off a healthful diet, and your perception of how thin you ought to be.

Once you have reached your ideal weight and believe you have control, you may want to include richer foods, such as dried fruits, nuts, seeds, avocados, olives, and soybeans (tofu or soy milk). Eventually, you may even choose to celebrate with traditional holiday favorites, like Thanksgiving turkey, Easter eggs, and birthday cake and ice cream.

BOOKS THAT PRESENT McDOUGALL RECIPES

The New McDougall Cookbook (Dutton, 1993)

The McDougall Program: 12 Days to Dynamic Health (Plume, 1991)

The McDougall Health-Supporting Cookbook, Volume II (New Win, 1986)

The McDougall Health-Supporting Cookbook, Volume I (New Win, 1985)

The McDougall Plan (New Win, 1983)

See the Appendix for specific recipes that fit the McDougall Program for Maximum Weight Loss from other books.

Are You Now Too Thin?

One of the most common concerns I hear from people who follow the McDougall Program faithfully is "I've lost too much weight."

Many people just think they're too thin when they're really not. For years, their mirrors have reflected an image of a much larger person. Now this new, thin body looks unfamiliar. Friends may ask, "Are you ill? You've lost so much weight." These friends may be truly concerned or they may have a sour-grapes attitude, longing to be just as trim. New friends will probably find you just the right size. "Too fat" and "too thin" are very subjective determinations.

If you are truly unhappy about your appearance, reversing the principles of the McDougall Program for Maximum Weight Loss may change the way you look. Add more flour products and cooked foods, and eat fewer green and yellow vegetables. Next add dried fruits. Finally add nuts, seeds, avocados, olives, and soybean products (including tofu). With the use of these high-fat plant foods, I could easily design a diet even higher in calories and fats than most Americans eat, and solve the problem of being too thin.

When you evaluate your diet, consider other lifestyle factors that may affect your weight. Exercise causes weight loss. Some people overdo physical activity, such as some long-distance runners, who can suffer the consequences of excess physical demands, including emaciation, anemia, and disturbances of menstrual cycles. In this case, less vigorous exercise may be a prudent choice.

Going On the Program Doesn't Mean Giving Up Tasty Eating

Cooking without oil and not eating meat and dairy products requires learning some new cooking methods and paying new attention to food combinations and to seasonings. I have included in Chapter 15 a section on cooking methods, as well as twenty-one days of sample menus for breakfast, lunch, dinner, and snacks as well. The recipes in Chapter 16 range from quick and easy to gourmet masterpieces. You'll find that learning this new approach to food sparks new interest in cooking and eating—it's actually a culinary adventure.

People enjoy foods that are familiar. Since a diet composed entirely of starches, vegetables, and fruits is new to most people, the McDougall Program for Maximum Weight Loss will require a period of adjustment. Give yourself that time and allow the adjustment to happen. You will find that these foods are not as unfamiliar as you might initially believe. In fact, they are old friends, elevated to a starring role. They can be dramatically enhanced by proper cooking and lively seasoning.

The maximum-weight-loss eating plan consists of many interesting foods and a great variety of flavors, aromas, colors, and textures. All of these can be brought to life with the use of favorite herbs, spices, salt, and even limited sugar. Within a week, you should not only be used to the diet, but enjoying your new foods.

Good eating is a pleasure not only because it satisfies our hunger but also because it stimulates our senses. There are three primary pleasures from food that nature has designed us to enjoy: the tastes of salt and sweetness, and the aroma of spice. We like sweet and salty tastes because we have taste buds for these flavors built in at the tip of the tongue. We respond to the aroma of food because of receptors in the nose. Much of food's pleasurable aromas come from herbs and spices, and from aromatic vegetables. Notable examples of these include mushrooms (cooked), onions, and garlic. In other words, a large part of what we enjoy about food comes from its seasonings. The maximum-weight-loss eating plan uses all of these pleasurable seasonings to delicious advantage.

You will soon realize that the only thing you have given up by going on the McDougall Program for Maximum Weight Loss is a lifetime battle with obesity.

CHAPTER 7

Women Are Slow Losers

Though it will come as no great surprise to many of my female readers, the fact is that men and women store and burn fat at different rates. Women, scientists have learned, accumulate fat more quickly than men, and burn it more slowly. This will confirm what many women have long suspected. Already I can hear perplexed voices saying, "I could have told scientists that a long time ago, and saved them a lot of effort."

Nevertheless, in this regard, we humans are right in step with the entire animal kingdom. For many reasons, some of which are still mysterious to scientists, female animals accumulate fat more quickly than male animals do, and they burn that fat more slowly than males. What all of this means is that women are at a disadvantage when it comes to losing weight. Moreover, if you are a woman and eat the standard American diet, your body actually works against you in your struggle to achieve normal weight. In fact, it's darn near impossible for a woman eating a typical American diet to keep that weight off.

Let me show you why.

Why Are Women Naturally Fatter?

Let's begin our discussion by acknowledging that the definition of "overweight" is, to some extent, cultural. To prove the point, we need only look at a few representative paintings of seventeenth-century Flemish artist Peter Paul Rubens, whose portraits of well-rounded women represented the epitome of female beauty during his time. Today Rubens's figures would be considered overweight, but the image of beauty he depicted has endured a lot longer than our current standard. On the other hand, obesity, which is defined as carrying 25 percent more than one's ideal weight, is objectively unhealthy and, by most definitions, unattractive.

Still, between our current standard of beauty and obesity lies a lot of adipose tissue, especially when it's on women.

A century ago, both Americans and Europeans regarded being slightly overweight as a sign of prosperity, particularly for women. A somewhat overweight woman was considered an asset to her family because, during times of scarcity, she could work longer on less food. It was recognized that body fat provides insulation from the cold and padding to protect the bones from hard surfaces, both good things to have when the work was hard and often performed outdoors. A little excess fat also accentuates attractive body curves, a nice characteristic when indoors.

Such cultural aesthetics, however, were more in line with biological necessities than our own standards of beauty are today. I am talking, of course, about childbearing. A woman's body must meet the demands of pregnancy and nursing, even during periods of food scarcity. Hence, nature has made it easier for women to accumulate fat and hold on to it tenaciously.

Metabolic Efficiency for Pregnancy

During pregnancy, a woman's appetite increases, prompting her to take in more calories and nutrients so that growth of the baby proceeds normally. But the extra nutrition also supports changes in a woman's own body, such as those in the uterus, placenta, and breasts. During the course of her pregnancy, a woman requires about two extra pounds of protein—in addition to her own biological needs—and an estimated 80,000 calories (an average of 300 extra calories a day). A woman's average weight gain during pregnancy on the standard American diet is 27.5 pounds. For women of normal weight, about eight of those pounds are fat, but heavier women tend to gain more. The hormone responsible for changes in appetite is probably progesterone, the so-called pregnancy hormone.

Nature has so perfectly designed women to give birth that they will produce healthy children even in times of food scarcity. For example, women living in underdeveloped countries where food supply may be short and food intake can decrease during pregnancy still bear normal, healthy children without difficulty. They manage this feat because their bodies increase metabolic efficiency during pregnancy. That means that a woman's body automatically decreases its resting metabolic rate and physical activity, both of which conserve energy.

Women Are Designed to Carry Extra Weight

Women are designed by nature to carry extra weight, and a woman's body is even more reluctant to give up its extra weight when exercised than a man's body is. For example, one study tested eight women who walked on a motorized treadmill. The women were placed in a special room called a whole-body calorimeter, which measures energy expenditure during exercise. As they walked, additional weights were added, up to 45 percent of each woman's body weight. For some, that meant carrying an additional sixty-six pounds. And they did it for fifteen minutes at a time.

The scientists wanted to know whether the women could carry some additional weight without actually raising the level of calories they burned. Remarkably, each of these women was able to carry at least 20 percent of her own body weight before she increased her energy expenditure. Thus, a woman weighing 100 pounds could carry an extra 20 pounds (or 20 percent of her weight) without increasing her energy consumption above the level she burned when walking without a load. Even though each woman was carrying a good deal of extra weight, her body reacted as if it weren't carrying the weight at all.

Again, we see nature's intention. A pregnant woman must be able to gain weight during her pregnancy while she efficiently carries a baby and additional supplies of nutrition within her body for nine months. You would think that all the extra weight of the baby would force a woman's body to burn more calories as exercise. But pregnancy changes the rules of the game, and in this sense, it is a feat that defies the conventional rules of nutrition and metabolism. However, for the non-pregnant woman, this means that the extra twenty pounds will be difficult to lose without extra effort.

This metabolic efficiency extends beyond pregnancy. In general, women have a lower resting metabolic rate than men, which means that they burn fewer calories to maintain basic life functions than men do. The differences are quite impressive: A small woman may need only 1,000 calories a day to maintain normal biological activities, a larger woman only 1,600. Men, on the other hand, need anywhere from 1,350 to 2,140 calories a day.*

Women's Specialized Fat Storage

Women's fat is even stored fat in different places than men's. This is done to ensure that calories (or supplies of energy) are available for pregnancy and lactation. Women have greater gluteal (on the buttocks) and femoral (on the upper leg) deposits. The fat is easily carried in these parts of the body. And hormones make these energy reserves accessible to the fetus and to the breasts on demand.

Another distinction between the sexes is that fat in men is deposited inside their abdominal cavity, while fat in women is

---

* Biologic activities are separate from physical activities. Since at least 1,000 calories are required to keep the heart beating, the lungs breathing, and the tissues alive, people claiming weight gain on 800 calorie diets are fooling only themselves.

deposited below the surface of the skin. Women also have larger fat cells than men.

Again, sex hormones produce these differences in fat distribution. Remarkably, when a woman passes menopause and estrogen levels decline, her fat stores begin to look and respond more like a man's. When men take estrogens as part of the treatment for prostate cancer they feminize their fat deposits.

Since excess fat deposits in women play a natural role in reproduction, they are likely to occur even with healthier eating practices. Excess fat accumulation in men does not occur for such innate reasons, and therefore is more likely a consequence of a rich diet and a lack of physical activity. As a result, obesity in men is associated with a greater likelihood of health problems. When doctors compare men and women with the same degree of relative body weight, men suffer more ill health: They have higher systolic and diastolic blood pressures, and higher levels of cholesterol, triglycerides, glucose, and insulin. On the other hand, women who have male-pattern weight—or abdominal fat—have the same increased health risks as men.

Abdominal fat is mobilized and burned more easily than fat around the hips and thighs—the places where women tend to accumulate fat. This is one reason why women lose extra fat more slowly than men. This explains too why women who add considerable weight to their hips and thighs during pregnancy have a much harder time losing it after childbirth. However, women who breast-feed speed their loss of excess hip and thigh fat.

What all of this means is that even when women are watching their diets, they are still likely to put on extra weight. This causes many women confusion and frustration, especially if they are counting calories and always suffering from hunger. "All I have to do is look at food to gain weight" is a common lament. Indeed, women are going to store some weight naturally no matter what they eat, but those who eat fatty foods are going to be overweight—by anyone's standards.

There are two ways to respond to this fact: either give up the effort to lose weight, as many women are doing today; or change the composition of your diet to the McDougall Program for Maximum Weight Loss and forget about dieting and weight loss. The McDougall Program will allow you to be naturally thin and attractive without effort.

That's what forty-six-year-old Susan Super of Juneau, Alaska, did. Susan adopted the McDougall Program for Maximum Weight Loss and dropped fifty pounds.

"I started on the McDougall Program when participating with my husband in the program at St. Helena Hospital. I realized that I had feasted enough in my lifetime. I went from a size 16 dress to a size 8. I have kept the weight off for three years now. It took me about eight months to lose 50 pounds. I don't need to lose any more; I'm a thin 120 pounds. [She is 5 feet 6 inches tall.] On the McDougall diet you can eat all you want, whenever you are hungry. You don't eat any animal products at all, which appeals to me for ethical reasons. I look so much better in clothes, can wear younger-looking styles, don't have to worry about horizontal stripes anymore. I look younger and more healthy. My skin is not as oily. My cholesterol went from a high of 191 to 119. I have more energy."

Working with Your Body's Efficiency

Now that you are aware of the superb efficiency of your female body and the important reasons for such a wondrous design, you can take steps necessary to lose undesired fat. Essentially, this means following the specific recommendations described in this book and putting a little more effort into your exercise program. No dieting—you are still expected to eat to the full satisfaction of your hunger drive while following these modifications to a starch-based diet and daily exercise.

As you will see in Chapter 9, which describes the exercise program, you needn't overdo exercise. We're talking about a lifetime commitment to health and optimal weight. Follow both the diet and the exercise program without starving yourself or following too strenuous an exercise regimen. This is not a torturous program: It is one that works with your nutritional and physical needs, not against them. The program is about harmony, not deprivation. In short, it is a program that will last.

Grace Telfer, a fifty-seven-year-old registered nurse and homemaker from St. Clairsville, Ohio, began the diet in 1989.

Within four months of starting the diet, she lost forty-seven pounds. She went through six dress sizes and lost four inches from her waist. Four years later (at the time of this writing), Grace was still on the diet and had never regained the weight she lost. Grace said she is fully satisfied with her diet—she follows it "about 99 percent of the time"—and is never hungry. "It is so simple that there is no reason to change anything. There is such a variety of foods that one never needs to be hungry or bored. I eat out less often than I used to, but I still eat out. If the restaurant will not prepare the food the way I want, I simply leave, but there have been very few problems."

When I asked Grace about her previous attempts at weight control, she gave me the usual Cook's tour of diets. "You name it, I've tried it—group therapy, Weight Limited, Weight Watchers, Cambridge, grapefruit diet, and any others that came along. I can't remember them all. I lost weight easily, but was bored, felt deprived, and gained it all back, and then some."

As for exercise, Grace is doing well. She walks or does aerobics for an hour a day five days a week. The combination of the diet and exercise has brought remarkable changes in her life—and her husband's!

"I've been healthy, but I feel even better now, and I'm more confident, and happier. To my surprise, my husband decided to try it himself, and has done better than me: He's lost fifty-five pounds, and has maintained it. He works twelve to fourteen hours a day, and exercises four times a week. Much appreciated benefits are he doesn't snore anymore, and has lost his big gut. I don't worry anymore about losing him to heart disease—his cholesterol was at one time 545, and is now 170."

Women are indeed slower losers than men, but that does not mean they cannot regain a youthful figure and good health. They simply must use the right method.

CHAPTER 8

Obesity Can Be Cured

Like many obese people, Linda Parker, thirty-nine, of Union City, California, had tried the standard approaches to weight loss and failed. She weighed more than 285 pounds and had all but given up hope of ever weighing less when she encountered the McDougall Program.

"I learned of this approach from a friend and started on the program October 6, 1991," Linda said. "It took six months to go from 285 to 160 pounds." At last count, she had lost 136 pounds on the McDougall Program and was still losing.

Linda advises people who are skeptical, "Tell yourself you are doing the program for twelve days only, following the guidelines in the book. After you go through the twelve days strictly, you will feel great and go on it forever. I have several friends whom I helped through your program, and they are doing well also. I also tell people that this program is not for everyone. You have to want to decide to feel good and take charge of your life."

Her only exercise is daily walking. That has been enough. "I have a new attitude, new clothes, and a new me," she said. "I am not tired and feel *great*! I no longer need allergy medication, iron, or Advil."

Nothing better illustrates the necessity for changing the

composition of the diet than obesity. Not only are obese people struggling against hunger and fat, like all overweight people, but they face an array of unique barriers to weight loss. Let's take a closer look.

Handicaps to Weight Loss: Obese People Do Not Eat More

A growing body of evidence suggests that obese people do not eat any more than lean people. Obese people may be unable to lose weight as easily as lean people because they have more efficient metabolisms. They need fewer calories to accomplish the same tasks. They may also be less active. The combination makes it virtually impossible for obese people to lose weight on the standard American diet—even when they count calories.

The validity of this evidence depends on the assumption that the obese people studied have accurately reported their intake of food and their activity levels. But if the evidence is accurate—and many people have suspected as much for decades—the principles of the McDougall Program for Maximum Weight Loss seem essential to obese people who want to lose weight.

Six scientific studies have found no significant difference in calorie intake between obese and nonobese populations. A review of five studies examining calorie differences between obese and nonobese people reported that the obese people ate significantly less than their nonobese peers. Four studies of obese adults, and five more of obese adolescents, reported that they consume significantly fewer calories than their nonobese counterparts.

This research implies that obese people require less energy to live and function than nonobese people. This may explain why the same activities in both groups cause smaller weight losses in the obese people than in the nonobese.

Inherited Efficiency

Most of human history has been marked by a struggle to find enough food. Our bodies have adapted to the condition of scarcity by making our cells work very efficiently. They do their work on the fewest possible calories. This has enabled us to survive in times of food shortages and famine.

Today most Americans have more than enough to eat. Hence, we take in more calories (especially fat calories) than are needed to conduct our lives, which ironically has turned our evolutionary advantage as human beings—our efficient metabolism—into a handicap. We are storing too many calories.

This is especially the case for some us who are blessed (or cursed, depending on how you look at it) with especially efficient cellular metabolism. Some research has demonstrated that this metabolic efficiency runs in families, obviously suggesting a genetic link. The weight of adopted children resembles that of their biological parents more than that of their adoptive parents.

Resting metabolic rate (RMR)—the rate at which you burn calories while resting—has been found to be passed along in families. This efficiency in obese people even extends to their ability to maintain body heat. Studies have shown that obese people burn fewer calories to maintain the same temperature than do nonobese people.

Other mysterious differences exist between obese people and nonobese. For example, the sight, sound, and smell of food elicit a small increase in blood insulin in people of normal weight and a much more pronounced increase in obese people. Even obese people who have reduced to normal weight have this exaggerated response. (Insulin causes fat to remain in fat cells and prevents its release. See Chapter 5 for more on insulin's role in weight loss.)

Indeed, the metabolic advantage of obese people turns against them even more when they attempt to lose weight.

The Dieter's Enhanced Efficiency

Obese people may be compounding their problems with their efforts to become thin. As I pointed out in Chapter 1, repeatedly restricting calories to lose excess fat trains the body to gain and hold on to calories efficiently, a vestige of an evolutionary adaptation to repeated famines. People develop a lower expenditure of energy at rest and during exercise. Consequently, they burn fewer calories, or less energy. Their intestines also become more efficient at absorbing foodstuffs. For an obese person with an already efficient system, these changes make weight loss even more difficult.

Economy of Activity

Obviously, obese people must work harder to carry around their larger bodies. It takes more energy for an obese person to walk or run a certain distance than it does a lean person. So you would think that if you got an obese person walking or running, he or she would have an advantage in losing weight, because it would be like walking or running with additional weights strapped on.

Interestingly, obese people frequently have been observed to have a certain economy of movement, which produces a lower calorie expenditure than that of lean people performing the same work. In a classic study of teenage women playing volleyball, the obese women had much less arm and leg movement during the game and expended fewer calories than the nonobese.

Too Many Fat Cells?

Another handicap in weight control is the relative number of fat cells in the body. Fat storage may be accomplished by an increase in the size of fat cells or in the number of fat cells in the tissues. The extremely obese show a marked increase in the number of fat cells. The number of fat cells can be determined in infancy; an overfed infant develops more fat cells, so that the overfeeding leads to a lifelong tendency to obesity. In adulthood, the fat cells become "sponges" for fat, filling themselves with triglycerides, or fatty acids, from high-fat meals. It follows that the more "sponges"—fat cells—you have, the faster the fat will be absorbed and the greater will be your tendency to hold on to the fat.

Inherited or Learned?

All of these factors point to possible genetic and developmental influences that may affect weight gain and loss. But before you lament your genes, take heart. You are not doomed to obesity, despite your experience with failed diets. There is more to this picture than what I have provided so far.

The truth is, characteristics of health and appearance that run in families are subject not only to genes but to family dietary patterns. These patterns influence our short- and long-term health and weight. They even extend to our pets: Fat dog owners tend to have fat dogs, but the cause is obviously not genetic. Fat husbands tend to have fat wives; in fact, the correlation between overweight spouses is as strong as that found between overweight parents and children. Proven environmental diseases, such as colon cancer, coronary artery disease, and adult-onset diabetes, all run in families—not necessarily because of genes, but because family members share the same dietary patterns. Simply put, you learn how to cook and what foods to like from your parents.

In fact, numerous studies have shown that there is a strong socioeconomic association among obese Americans that cannot be explained by genetics. People with lower incomes are more likely to be obese, especially women. No one is saying that the people of this socioeconomic strata are genetically related. Moreover, there are countries where obesity is almost unknown, like China. Yet when Chinese emigrate to the United States and give up their starch-based diet of rice and vegetables, they lose their immunity to obesity and their thin, healthy appearance. Many Chinese-Americans become overweight and ill when they adopt the rich American diet.

Genetic factors do indeed play a role in the efficiency and speed of metabolism. But these factors only make those with efficient bodies more vulnerable to weight gain when they eat a high-fat, low-carbohydrate diet.

Recent research on adults and children clearly shows the problem: Obese people consume foods higher in fat and lower in carbohydrate than nonobese people, even if the total calories are the same. Fatty snacks, such as chips and packaged cookies, were reported favorites of obese children, whereas the nonobese liked high-carbohydrate snacks like Popsicles and soft drinks.

According to obesity experts, although genetic factors may explain much of the individual variations in fatness within a society whose members are exposed to a similar diet, environmental influences must be invoked to account for the differences in fatness that occur between societies whose characteristic diets, activity levels, and attitudes concerning physical appearance differ. And when the two possibilities, genetic inheritance versus educational transmission, are compared, obesity is more of a learned disorder.

Overcoming Handicaps

You are not trapped in an inescapable situation. Your answer is the McDougall Program for Maximum Weight Loss. You will overcome your minor handicaps. After a few weeks or months, you will have control of your weight and be just as trim as people from trim families. You can do this without dieting—you will satisfy your hunger as long as you follow the starch-based diet and do some daily exercise. It's as easy as that.

Orrenn H. DuBow of New York City, forty-six years old, lost ninety-four pounds; Francis Schaefer of Glenburn, North Dakota, sixty-seven years old, lost seventy pounds; Paul V. Capps of Durham, North Carolina, thirty-seven years old, lost eighty-nine pounds.

Orrenn DuBow learned of the McDougall Program from our first book, *The McDougall Plan*, which she read in 1987. "I started on it immediately," Orrenn said. "My reason was that I had reached 220 pounds, had extremely high blood lipids, hypertension, and I looked like a tub. I have now been on the starch-based diet for the past seven years. I weigh 130 pounds. This change took six to seven months. I went from a size 24 dress to a 7/8. My waist was forty-two inches; it's now twenty-six. I look better than I did at twenty. As time goes on I adhere even more strictly to the plan, because when I'm faithful the benefits are striking."

Francis Schaefer was listening to the radio in Phoenix when he heard me being interviewed. Two months later Francis was diagnosed with diabetes. He remembered the McDougall Program and began it immediately. "In seven months I lost seventy pounds, my waist went from forty-two to thirty-eight inches, and I've stayed with the program for six years.

"My blood sugar has become normal; my cholesterol dropped to 127. I have stopped taking all medication. I'm able to take care of my five-acre yard, a garden, and a half acre of trees."

Paul Capps "just happened to pick up *The McDougall Program* in a local bookstore and started thumbing through it. In two days, I started the diet, and lost the weight in a little over nine months. I now weigh 180 pounds. I have lost 89 pounds and twelve inches off my waist and I eat a lot more food than before."

Many of the people who come to the McDougall Program were struggling with obesity and the false belief that the condition could not be cured. Chronic obesity can be cured, and you don't have to starve yourself to do it. All you need to do is change the composition of your diet to the foods that provide lots of carbohydrates and very little fat.

CHAPTER 9

An Exercise Program
You Can Live With

On paper, losing weight is pretty simple: You either decrease your intake of calories (specifically, calories from fat), or increase your expenditure of calories, or both. But as you have seen, unless you follow the right diet, your chances of losing weight and keeping it off are pretty small.

As with diet, there are many misconceptions about exercise. Images of sweat and strain and clichés like "no pain, no gain" make exercise seem more like torture than fun. Contrary to what many people believe, however, you don't have to do a lot of exercise to gain tremendous benefit. A simple walk in the park at least four times a week—preferably every day—will provide all the exercise you need, as long as you walk long enough and at a brisk pace. But as you will see, there are lots of enjoyable ways to exercise, and none of them has to be torturous.

On the McDougall Program for Maximum Weight Loss, you can and will lose lots of weight from the diet alone. But when you couple a little exercise with the dietary program, the weight loss is easier and faster. Also, exercise helps control your appetite and therefore helps you stick with the diet. Moreover, you get numerous health benefits from moderate exercise, including the fact that you will be shedding body fat and replacing it with muscle. Not a bad deal.

Despite all the evidence proving how beneficial exercise is for body and mind, only 37 percent of all Americans regularly exercise, according to a recent Harris Poll. Among other reasons, our tendency to conserve energy, and thus hold on to calories, also helps us resist exercise.

Consider whether you prefer to:

• Drive short distances rather than walk
• Search, then sometimes wait, for the closest parking spot rather than take a few extra steps
• Ride the elevator rather than walk the stairs
• Lie and sit rather than stand
• Walk to meetings rather than run

Conservation of energy favors human survival because of the historical vicissitudes of our food supply. In other words, when we exercise, we are actually working against some fundamental urge within ourselves to adopt a sedentary lifestyle.

Diet and Exercise: A Healthy Marriage

Diet and exercise are an interesting couple. One makes the other more effective. Consequently, they have a greater impact on your life when you use both rather than relying on one or the other. Let me explain.

If you eat a low-fat diet and exercise, you will burn more calories than if you just eat a low-fat diet. The result will be greater weight loss.

Interestingly, the evidence demonstrates that those who diet and exercise tend to stick to their dietary regimens longer. Also, more of these people enjoy permanent weight loss than those who diet but do not exercise.

Exercise accomplishes this in several ways. The research shows that those who exercise experience improved psychological health and greater self-esteem than those who don't. Exercise is associated with improvement in mood, feelings of well-being, a reduction in anxiety and stress, and even euphoria. People feel personally empowered by exercise.

Exercise also changes brain chemistry. After only twenty minutes of running, the brain secretes elevated levels of beta-endorphins, morphine-like compounds that create the "natural high" runners frequently talk about. This affects the mind in many ways, but among the more salient is the fact that even mild depression is relieved with exercise. These positive psychological benefits may prevent relapses to the old eating habits, especially since a positive self-image encourages more positive and life-supportive behaviors.

Also, as you start to feel better thanks to your diet and exercise program, the positive cycle encourages its own continuation. This is especially true of people who are very overweight. For one thing, they burn more calories from any form of weight-bearing exercise—such as walking or jogging—because they must carry more weight per step than people who are trimmer. Thus, overweight people expend more energy and experience greater weight loss during the same exercise periods than those who weigh less. These good results encourage greater compliance, which leads to even better results. In this way, the positive cycle is perpetuated.

On a high-carbohydrate diet, people are found to feel less tension, depression, and anger when they exercise as compared to people who exercise on a low-carbohydrate diet.

Of course, besides these benefits, significant physical activity reduces other risk factors related to obesity. For example, exercise lowers blood pressure; raises HDL ("good") cholesterol; lowers triglycerides; and increases insulin sensitivity, thus reducing diabetics' dependence on medication. All of these improvements reduce the risk of heart attacks and strokes.

Exercise improves the efficiency of your heart, meaning that it is able to pump more blood per beat and rest longer between beats.

Medical Screening for Exercise

Before you exercise, you should know the condition of your health, especially your cardiovascular system. That requires a blood pressure test, a cholesterol test, and an electrocardiogram (EKG). People who are moderately obese—weighing up to 130 percent of ideal weight, based on life insurance tables—but have no other health problems (including high cholesterol, hypertension, cigarette smoking, abnormal EKG, or heart trouble) have no greater medical risk when exercising than people in the general population. However, you must know your risk factors before you begin such an exercise program. The older you are, the more important such a medical evaluation is.

A treadmill stress test may be helpful in providing some reassurance that you can safely handle a certain level of exercise. However, these tests have not been found to reduce the risk of death. You should know your blood pressure and cholesterol when starting an exercise program; they will give you reliable indications of the state of your health. The higher these values, the greater your risk.

Warning: Change Your Diet Before You Exercise

The richer your diet, the greater your risk of suffering a heart attack or stroke during exercise. Cemeteries are filled with people who have died of heart attacks before, during, and after completing a triumphant endurance run. Your risk increases if you fail to change your diet *before* beginning an exercise program.

Fats and oils in the American diet cause red blood cells to adhere to one another, resulting in a 20 percent reduction in the amount of oxygen carried by the blood to the tissues. This depletion of the oxygen-carrying capacity of the blood is especially critical to the heart, which is one of the muscles most stressed during exercise and thus requires increased oxygen. Insufficient oxygen and nutrients to the heart muscle, coupled with inadequate waste removal, can cause chest pain and may contribute to a heart attack and dangerous heartbeat irregularities (arrhythmias).

Most importantly, animal fats cause the blood to form clots, thus significantly increasing your risk of heart attack. When you consume (saturated) animal fats, the blood-clotting elements known as platelets become more adhesive—they stick together more easily. Also, the blood-clotting proteins become more active. These changes cause the blood to suddenly form clots, in a process known as thrombosis. When the clotting occurs in the heart artery, it is called a coronary thrombosis. For doctors, the term "coronary thrombosis" is synonymous with "heart attack."

However, your circulation, and the dangerous blood-clotting tendencies, begin to improve within five days of following the McDougall Program for Maximum Weight Loss. This means that the blood and oxygen supply to all tissues will be more dependable and more abundant. Such an improvement in circulation will affect every aspect of your health.

Therefore, people at risk of heart disease should eat well for several days before beginning an exercise program.

What to Do Before You Exercise

Besides following a healthful diet, you should spend ten to twenty minutes warming up before exercising. This should include gentle stretching exercises, which prepare the muscles for their workout. You should also start out at a relaxed pace and then increase your speed as your body adjusts to the increased demands. Finally, you should finish your workout with a cool-down period that includes a short stroll and some gentle stretching. These measures will keep your muscles more limber and prevent them from excessively tightening after your workout. Your clothing should be loose and comfortable so that your skin can breathe and your body can regulate its temperature.

Before we get to specific types of exercises, let's look briefly at how you can benefit from exercise.

Weight-Losing Reasons to Exercise

1. Exercise Burns Calories

Most of the calories you eat each day are used to run your life-sustaining machinery, such as the heart, lungs, brain, and liver. These functions are clumped together in a category called resting metabolic rate (RMR). When you increase physical movement, your calorie expenditure exceeds these basic demands. That's what happens during exercise: You require your body to do more than merely survive. Once you begin to exercise, fat is used by the body for energy, which begins to decrease your weight.

Calories Burned per Minute During Exercise
(based on speed of walking and body weight)

Weight (lb)							
	100	140	180	220	260	300	340
Speed (mph)							
2	2	2.8	3.6	4.4	5.2	6.0	6.9
2.5	2.3	3.3	4.2	5.1	6.0	6.9	7.9
3	2.6	3.7	4.7	5.8	6.8	7.8	8.9
3.5	2.9	4.1	5.3	6.4	7.6	8.8	10.0
4	3.2	4.6	5.8	7.1	8.4	9.7	11.0

Data from American College of Sports Medicine, *Guidelines for Exercise Testing and Prescription*, 3d ed. (Philadelphia: Lea & Febiger, 1986).

2. Calories Continue to Burn After Exercise

You may have been discouraged by reading charts that tell you that only 100 calories are expended in walking one mile—that's the caloric equivalent of only an ounce of cheese or a medium potato. (If nothing else, these charts help us realize the importance of food choices, especially how easy it is to put on weight and how difficult it can be to take it off.) Fortunately, exercise increases energy expenditure for many hours after your workout. Stored glycogen that was held inside the muscles must be replaced; also, muscle tissue that was broken down during exercise must be repaired after the workout is finished. Both of these processes require postexercise calories.

Even more important, exercise increases your resting metabolic rate, which means that your cells continue to burn energy at a higher rate even while you are sitting down. One study showed that after exercising for eighty minutes, people experienced a 15 percent increase in energy expenditure for twelve hours. This postexercise rise in resting metabolic rate is easily lost, however. All you have to do is stop exercising for three days and the higher RMR returns to its slower rate.

Sustained postexercise energy expenditure is seen only with aerobic exercises such as walking, running, bicycling, dancing, basketball, tennis, and cross-country skiing.

3. Exercise Counteracts Plateaus

As you saw in Chapter 2, whenever you diet, your body shifts into survival mode, which slows metabolism and stores calories. This is experienced by dieters as a plateau, or a point at which they can no longer lose weight. This is usually a very discouraging period, and many people simply give up any hope of weight loss. The consequence is clear: Weight loss creates adaptive changes that retard further weight loss.

However, by speeding metabolic rate, exercise counteracts these plateaus and assures the dieter continued weight loss.

4. Exercise Suppresses Appetite

Exercise is commonly believed to increase appetite, but in fact it has been shown to decrease appetite, or keep it at the previous level. Five of the seven studies done on the relation between calorie intake and activity reported a decrease in calorie intake with exercise training, or very small changes in calorie intake with training. In those overweight people for whom exercise increases appetite, studies have shown that any increase in calorie consumption is less than the calories burned. Consequently, there is a net loss of calories and a loss of weight.

Thus, the most common effect of exercise is to depress appetite mildly. Exercise often readjusts the mechanisms of hunger, sometimes referred to as the "appestat," which causes further weight reduction and trimness.

In one recent study published in the *American Journal of Clinical Nutrition*, twenty men and women of normal weight were followed during consecutive five-day periods in which each group exercised during one period and did not exercise during the next. Calorie intake in men increased during the exercise period by an average of 208 calories per day. However, because of the increased physical activity, they each used an extra 596 calories daily, on average. Consequently, they lost 388 calories of fat each day because of the exercise. The women did not increase their food intake during exercise, but they did burn an extra 382 calories a day.

5. Exercise Reduces Insulin

As was discussed in Chapter 5, elevated insulin keeps fat from being burned. Increasing physical activity lowers the body's insulin, thus allowing fat to leave the fat cells to be burned as fuel.

6. Exercise Protects and Increases Muscle Mass

Muscle is a highly active tissue. It burns lots of calories just to keep itself alive. Once they begin to work, muscles burn even more calories. Fat cells, however, are more inert, requiring relatively few calories to survive. Therefore, even a resting muscular body uses more calories than a pudgy one.

Weight-loss programs often cause a loss of muscle and, once the diet is dropped, an increase in fat. Loss of muscle mass is especially great when a dieter uses a powdered protein regimen, such as Optifast and the Cambridge Diet.

Exercise helps to protect the muscle during dieting. In one study, adults were divided into three groups: One group reduced their food intake by 500 calories a day, but did not exercise. The second group increased physical activity to expend 500 calories a day; the third group reduced calories by 250 and increased expenditure by 250 calories. All lost similar amounts of weight. The group who dieted without exercise lost a considerable amount of muscle mass, however, while those with exercise in their program lost more fat and maintained more muscle mass.

You can double or triple your muscle mass with exercise. However, by staying inactive and gorging yourself on rich foods, you can increase the amount of fat in your body a thousandfold. The potential for ruination is much greater.

Frequency of Exercise

You'll need to exercise three days or more per week to change your body weight and to reduce the amount of fat your body carries. The more frequently you exercise, the more easily you will lose.

Weight loss is directly related to the work done. A 200-pound man who walks one mile burns 100 calories; if he runs that mile, he burns 150 calories; if he bicycles a mile, he uses 54 calories. However, people usually bicycle for more than a mile at a time, so bicycling can be a wonderful form of exercise.

No Pain, Yes Gain

Avoid the philosophy of "no pain, no gain." Exercise performed in the wrong way, or too vigorously for the shape you're in, may cause injury, or worse. That "drive yourself over the cliff" attitude isn't necessary.

While exercising, your muscles derive energy from a combination of carbohydrate and stored fat. When you are exercising at 60 percent of capacity—not a full-throttle workout by any means—you are deriving about half your energy from carbohydrate and the other half from fat. But as you increase the intensity of your workout—say, to 90 percent of muscle capacity—you get your energy almost entirely from carbohydrate. In other words, the harder levels of intensity burn little fat.

Thus, to burn fat, your exercise program should be one of moderate and sustained exercise. When the program becomes too strenuous, you'll exhaust yourself without burning much fat.

Self-Test

The best way to gauge the correctness of your exercise level is to keep track of your breathing. You should be able to carry on a conversation with someone while you exercise. If you exceed your optimal levels, you will not be able to talk while you exercise; at that point, slow down, catch your breath, and resume a more moderate pace. Check yourself periodically by seeing whether you can talk comfortably while you are walking, running, or performing some other exercise.

There are also the standard formulas for those who are interested in measuring their heart rates during exercise. In order to improve your cardiovascular and muscular fitness, your heart must beat at 60 to 90 percent of its maximum rate, according to the American College of Sports Medicine. To know your maximum heart rate, subtract your age from 220. If you are forty, your maximum heart rate is 180. In order to achieve a training level of exercise, you should be able to get your heart rate up between 108 (60 percent of 180) beats per minute, to a maximum of 162 (90 percent of 180) beats per minute, and keep it there for fifteen to twenty minutes. That will ensure that you are improving your overall conditioning. I do not like this formula as much as the conversation test because it promotes unnecessary overexertion. I recommend that you use the conversation test as a standard measure and the heart-rate test as a backup.

Make the time you exercise fun. If you enjoy exercise, it will become a habit.

Add Time Rather Than Intensity

It is safer and more effective to add time to your exercise than to increase the intensity. Adding ten minutes to a thirty-minute exercise session will burn 33 percent more calories.

To achieve effective weight loss, about 300 calories should be expended per session. That means that you need forty to sixty minutes of low-intensity walking, swimming, or bicycling to burn 300 calories. Twenty to thirty minutes of moderate to vigorous running will do the same.

Obviously, the length and intensity of your workout will determine how much energy you expend. But the source of that energy is different, depending on the type of exercise you perform.

During short, intense exercise periods, as with weight lifting, energy is provided from the stores of glycogen already present in your muscles.

During aerobic training, energy is needed over a longer period, requiring that prolonged energy and oxygen flow to the muscles from the blood. In the process, the muscles use fatty acids present in the bloodstream. The more physically trained your muscles become, the better they are at using fats. In this way, regular exercise prevents obesity and helps you reduce weight.

The longer you exercise, the more the fuel comes from fat stores. An extreme example of prolonged, strenuous exercise is the marathon. During the early stages of competition, muscle glycogen furnishes 90 to 95 percent of energy, while fat provides 10 percent or less. As the run continues, an increasing fraction of the energy is obtained from fats and a decreasing fraction from carbohydrates, so that near the end of the twenty-six miles as much as 95 percent of the runner's energy is derived from fat. Therefore, longer periods of exercise can be expected to produce more loss of fat from fatty tissues.

Begin Slowly and Increase Gradually

Start your exercise program slowly to avoid injury, exhaustion, pain, and discouragement. You should not be suffering from chest pains (angina), leg pains (claudication), or other body aches and pains. When you finish your exercise, you should feel better than when you started, not worse. As your fitness improves, gradually increase your exercise level. An out-of-shape beginner may do well with ten minutes of daily walking on a flat surface the first week. You can increase the length of time you exercise by five minutes each week until you are exercising forty to sixty minutes.

Exercise Just Before Meals

As I mentioned, exercise tends to suppress appetite. In overweight people, even small increases in appetite do not result in an increase in food consumption equal to the amount of calories lost. Consequently, you will experience a net loss of calories from exercise.

To take full advantage of the hunger-suppressing effects of exercise, you should exercise before meals whenever possible. Studies have shown that the appetite-suppressing effects of exercise are increased with the intensity of the exercise, and also when the meal comes close to the end of the exercise period. Food intake has been reduced in preschool children by changing recess from after lunch to before. Animal studies support the assertion that the appetite-suppressing effects of exercise are increased with the intensity of the workout, and that animals consume less when the meal is fed closer to the end of the exercise period.

Aerobics: The Best Kind of Exercise

Continuous activities that use the larger muscle groups—the legs and back, for example—are ideal for weight loss. Walking, running, cycling, and swimming are not only enjoyable but

highly efficient ways to lose weight. Tennis, basketball, rac-
quetball, and cross-country skiing are highly aerobic and excellent weight-loss exercises. Studies have shown that each of
these exercises is equally effective in reducing fat and changing
body composition (muscle versus fat), as long as the duration,
frequency, and intensity of the exercise are similar.

Your physical condition must be carefully considered when
you plan an exercise program. People with arthritis may be restricted in the exercises they can perform. In the extreme, they
may be limited to exercises with hand weights done in a wheel-
chair. Those who suffer from arthritis and those who are extremely obese may be able to protect the joints in their lower
extremities by doing various aerobic exercises in a swimming
pool. The water supports their bodies and eliminates much of
the shock to the joints of exercise. If you exercise in chin-deep
water, water aerobics can reduce your body weight by as much
as 90 percent. Water aerobics make a wonderful way to get a
workout.

The Benefits of Weight Training

Weight training is no longer just for bodybuilders. Research
is showing that people well into their nineties can benefit from
strength and flexibility training using weights. Below is just a
partial list of the benefits. Weight training can:

Build a stronger body
Build a shapelier body
Strengthen ligaments
Improve bone density (thus protecting against osteoporosis)
Help prevent musculoskeletal injury
Elevate metabolism
Increase stamina
Elevate blood levels of HDL cholesterol (thus protecting
    against heart disease)

Many athletes believe that because strength-building exercise "tears down" skeletal muscle tissue, there is a greater dietary need for protein, but this has not been demonstrated

by scientific research. In fact, the animals with the biggest muscles—hippopotamuses, horses, and elephants—eat grass and other plant matter, not the muscles of other animals. Generally, animals that eat other animals—cats, for example—are relatively small among the animal kingdom.

All the protein needed to grow large muscles is present in vegetable foods. Vegetables provide two to four times the protein anyone would need during any activity. Scientific studies tell us we need 2.5 percent of our calories in the form of protein. The World Health Organization has added a safety margin to protein requirements and says that we need 5 percent of our calories in the form of protein.

But let's look at how much protein vegetables offer.

Potatoes provide 11 percent protein; corn, 12 percent; oranges, 8 percent; cauliflower, 40 percent. And all of it is complete protein, meaning that these foods provide all the essential amino acids. When you add up all the protein-free sugar and fat calories most people eat, you will find that the American diet is about 12 percent protein, which is about the same as the McDougall Program for Maximum Weight Loss. If you still think you need more protein, choose beans, peas, and lentils, which provide 28 percent of their calories from protein, just like beef.

As I explained earlier, all that excess protein has a variety of negative effects on the body.

Spot Reduction Doesn't Work

Spot reduction is the use of certain exercises to remove fat from specific places on the body—doing sit-ups to reduce fat in the abdomen, for example, perhaps with the hope that the extra weight on the female bust will remain. Unfortunately for all you spot reducers, the research doesn't support this notion. One study found no difference in fat content or thickness of the right and left forearms of high-performance tennis players, who are doing high-intensity spot exercises continually.

Exercise stimulates the mobilization of fat from fat deposits throughout the body. The areas of greatest accumulation probably do lose the most fat. But the goal is to lose total fat.

Cellulite on the hips and thighs is a frequent site for spot-reduction exercises. However, obese subjects have been shown to lose fat in these areas only as quickly as in the rest of the body.

Your New Daily Exercise Plan

1. Get up half an hour earlier each day, or skip a TV program to do a specific exercise. Set a time, pick out your exercise clothes, and do it with commitment.

2. Make exercise a part of each day. Park your car farther from work or shopping areas; use the stairs whenever possible, rather than the elevator or escalator. Climbing uses more energy per minute than almost any other activity. Stand a little longer, rather than sit.

3. Choose an activity that you have always enjoyed and do it at least four times per week. Among the most popular are walks in the park, neighborhood, or woods; bicycle riding; tennis; swimming; water aerobics; and weight training at home. These activities cost little or nothing, and each of them will add quality and enjoyment to your life.

4. Sometimes purchasing equipment helps to motivate, such as a stair-climbing machine, a treadmill, cross-country ski equipment, a stationary cycle, or Nautilus equipment.

5. Invest in a membership in a YMCA, YWCA, or health and fitness club. Most colleges and universities offer surprisingly inexpensive health and fitness programs. Many of them have sliding-scale rates so that they can fit into most people's budgets.

6. Ask a friend to become your exercise partner. Often partners can help motivate each other, especially on days when one feels a little lazy.

7. Go dancing, a great aerobic (and romantic) exercise. There are swing dancing, contra dancing, and square

dancing clubs all over the country, and they cost little or nothing.

8. Join a walking or hiking club. Hiking clubs make for social walking. Also, such clubs often take special walks in beautiful parts of the country. It's a great way to get out, lose weight, and make friends.

9. Check with your local adult-education program for exercise programs.

10. Keep an exercise journal. By keeping a record of how much you've exercised, or the distance you walked or ran that day, you will be able to see how much your body is changing. Include your plan for exercise and weight loss and your conditioning goals. Periodically assess your fitness by monitoring your heart rate and your weight and having your cholesterol and blood pressure checked. Reward yourself with a new suit of clothes when you have reached a goal.

With each new demand, your body will be forced to lose fat and build muscle, so that you can go on walking, bicycling, swimming, running, climbing mountains, or dancing the night away. If you never ask your body to do better, you may never experience its miraculous potential for good looks and top performance.

CHAPTER 10

Alcohol, Coffee, and Your Weight

If you use alcohol, coffee, or weight-reducing drugs, you'll want to understand their effects on your health and appearance. Anyone who has drunk coffee or alcohol realizes that they have their attractions, which of course is the reason they're so popular. However, for many people, especially heavy users, the overall impact of alcohol or coffee detracts from the quality of life. I do not recommend the use of either, though some of the information that follows may be incorrectly interpreted by readers with a narrow perspective as a partial endorsement.

Alcohol Is Calorie-Concentrated

The average American over the age of fourteen consumes 2.65 gallons of pure (absolute) alcohol per year. Alcohol provides 7 calories per gram and 210 calories per ounce. In calories alone, that amounts to 71,232 calories per person per year. If all those calories were converted to fat, more than twenty pounds would be added per year on average to each person in the country. Since a third of the population doesn't drink, the actual calories-to-fat formula would put an additional twenty-eight pounds of weight per year on the average person who does drink.

Alcohol's Contribution to Obesity

A glass of wine or other alcoholic beverage contributes only seven calories per gram of alcohol, but alcohol can contribute to weight gain in several ways. Alcohol accelerates the absorption of sugar from the intestine, increasing the level of insulin in the body. By activating an enzyme called lipoprotein lipase (LPL), insulin causes fat cells to accumulate fat. Insulin also blocks the breakdown of fat from these same cells, keeping them, and you, plump.

More important than the calories and metabolic effects, alcohol changes what you eat and how much by relieving behavioral inhibitions. Alcohol removes the self-control required to tolerate hunger, which obviously works against your efforts at dieting. The best of intentions to stay away from fatty foods can be foiled by a couple of drinks.

Alcohol Itself Is Not Fattening

The calorie contribution of alcohol is complex and does not necessarily lead to obesity. In fact, many of the heaviest drinkers are quite trim. Drinking women especially have been found to be lighter than nondrinkers.

In one study, fifty-six alcoholics were fed an adequate diet of 2,600 calories a day and an additional 1,800 calories of alcohol (about sixteen ounces of distilled spirits) in a hospital setting. No greater weight gain was observed in these subjects than in those who did not receive the supplement of alcohol. In another study, 2,000 calories of alcohol added to an adequate diet resulted in no weight gain, but 2,000 calories of chocolate did cause subjects to gain weight.

Alcohol displaces other calories derived from the diet; it is also burned immediately as energy, or as heat. The process of turning alcohol into fat requires significant amounts of energy. Rather than waste such energy, the body burns off the excess calories as heat; so alcohol does not turn to fat, despite the added calories.

By providing these calories, however, alcohol prevents body fat from being burned, leaving fat in the adipose tissue. Thus, your attempts to lose weight are foiled by alcohol. When your diet consists of significant amounts of fat and alcohol, the calories from alcohol will be used for your daily physical and metabolic needs, while the fat will be stored in fatty tissues. The most efficient immediate use of dietary fat is simply to transport it to the fat cells.

The use of alcohol as part of a high-carbohydrate, low-fat diet will not encourage weight gain, because both of these kinds of calories will be burned as heat if consumed in excess of daily needs, rather than be stored as fat. In fact, replacing carbohydrate with alcohol will actually result in weight loss, because the metabolism of alcohol requires energy, thereby increasing energy expenditure.

For those drinkers who are unwilling to quit but are concerned about body weight and health, a low-fat, high-carbohydrate diet is especially important. Most people who continue to drink alcohol will stay trim, and those who need to will lose excess body fat on this healthful diet. Scientific evidence also suggests that common complications of excess drinking—such as fatty infiltration of the liver, alcoholic hepatitis, cirrhosis, and malnutrition—will be uncommon in drinkers who follow a starch-based diet with vegetables and fruits.

"Coffee Keeps Me Thin"

Coffee consumption usually encourages fat loss. The chemical compounds in coffee, including caffeine, suppress your appetite. For many people, coffee also causes nausea, which dampens appetite and eventually leads to weight loss. The appetite-suppressing effects can be powerful enough to cause anorexia with profound weight loss—to the point of becoming a life-threatening illness.

It has been known since 1915 that caffeine ingestion increases metabolic rate. In fact, two cups of coffee will increase metabolism significantly for at least three hours.

The amount of fat in the bloodstream doubles after caffeine is consumed, the result of fat being released from the fat cells. These fats are eventually burned away. This fat-burning effect of coffee is primarily due to the caffeine, and is greater in people of normal weight than in those who are obese.

Caffeine increases the loss of energy by heat production, a process known as thermogenesis. In one study, 100 milligrams of caffeine (one cup of regular coffee) caused the metabolic rate to increase by 3 to 4 percent over the next 150 minutes. If the dose of caffeine was repeated every two hours all day long (for twelve hours), the amount of energy expended increased by 8 to 11 percent. The net effect was an increase of 150 calories expended in lean people and 79 calories in postobese subjects (people who had previously been obese but were now of normal weight). Thus, the amount of coffee consumed by an average drinker can have a important effect on the energy balance and may promote weight loss. Losing 150 calories a day could translate into a pound of fat lost every twenty-four days.

Coffee stimulates the sympathetic nervous system, which depresses insulin activity and further contributes to weight loss. Caffeine also causes hyperventilation, which burns off more calories through the muscular work of respiration.

The Fattening Coffee Break

People who drink coffee have also been found to eat greater quantities of foods that are loaded with calories, cholesterol, and fat than non-coffee drinkers. Actually, a variety of excesses in behavior are commonly found in the same person. Overweight people tend to drink more coffee; eat fewer starches, vegetables, and fruits; and drink more alcohol. Although coffee has no calories, each teaspoon of sugar adds sixteen calories, and each tablespoon of creamer adds another twenty to forty calories. And for many people, a coffee break is not complete without a roll or a jelly doughnut.

Coffee can also cause many people to take in more food in an attempt to relieve the irritation of the stomach lining caused by the drink's many chemicals. This burning sensation of "acid indigestion" is perceived as hunger. Most daily coffee drinkers have learned that food will absorb much of the excess acid produced by the stomach as a result of the coffee, and will soothe the pain of indigestion.

Decaffeinated coffee causes the same amount of acid production, as well as stomach and intestinal distress, as regular coffee. Since decaffeinated coffee lacks the weight-reducing benefits of caffeinated coffee, it might be expected to lead to greater weight gain.

Coffee Used as Weight-Loss Therapy

Coffee and other sources of caffeine, alone or combined with other ingredients, have been used as effective weight-loss aids. Ephedrine, a natural drug widely available in a variety of forms but most often as a tea, is commonly used with caffeine. Taking Ephedrine increases heat production and metabolic rate by direct stimulation of the tissues and by increasing the activity of the sympathetic nervous system (norepinephrine). Ephedrine occurs naturally in plants and has been used in China for more than 5,000 years. Ephedrine teas can be purchased in natural-food stores, but the dose is difficult to determine and depends on many variables. These teas are sold as Mormon's tea, desert tea, Mauhuang, and Ephedra Sinica.

A combination of ephedrine and caffeine has produced weight loss as effectively as powerful prescription diet pills such as diethylpropion (brand name Tenuate). One study compared the effects of Tenuate and ephedrine-with-caffeine on obese patients. After twelve weeks, the average weight loss for 108 obese patients was nearly 18 pounds, using 120 milligrams of ephedrine and 300 milligrams of caffeine. Those taking 75 milligrams of diethylpropion (Tenuate) a day lost 18.5 pounds; the group being given a placebo lost 9 pounds.

A Price to Be Paid

Coffee is the most popular beverage in Western society, and for good reason: It's one of the last legal highs (along with alcohol and tobacco). It stimulates you to be keener and more alert. Unfortunately, side effects may lead to health problems, including higher cholesterol, indigestion, and diarrhea. Caffeine is present in significant amounts in coffee (103 milligrams in 6 ounces); high-caffeine teas (less than 100 milligrams in 6 ounces); instant coffee (57 milligrams in 6 ounces); tea (36 milligrams in 6 ounces); and colas (40 milligrams in 12 ounces).

Both caffeine and ephedrine are potent stimulants. They raise blood pressure and heart rate, cause irregularities in heartbeat, and dilate bronchial airways. People with heart disease or high blood pressure and those on medication (especially for hypertension or depression) should avoid these stimulants. Taking enough of these pills to cause weight loss would likely also cause most people significant side effects, and therefore cannot be recommended.

CHAPTER 11

Practical Ways of Managing Emotions

All of us, from time to time, eat purely because of emotional need. We reward ourselves with food; we celebrate our successes with a big meal; at times, we even use food to help us relax. Such behaviors arise partly out of tradition—secular and religious holidays incorporate food as part of ritual—and partly because we know instinctively that food has biological and psychological effects on us. It is precisely because food has such effects on us that it can be abused, especially by those who are chronically depressed.

Severe depression that requires medical attention is present in as much as 6 percent of the population. But many more people suffer from less severe depression, which still interferes with their lives. In other words, depression is a major health problem, and some studies suggest that it's getting worse.

I want to offer a couple of helpful tools to those who eat—or overeat—when they are depressed or emotionally low. I am not saying that every overweight person does this; nor am I saying that a majority of overweight people are depressed. But some people who are struggling with overweight do, indeed, overeat because they are suffering emotionally. There are safe, effective ways of dealing with depression. The first is diet; the second is exercise; the third is sleep management; and the fourth is mood-altering drugs. Drugs should be used only under a doctor's care. Exercise is discussed elsewhere in the book. In this chapter, I'd like to focus on the ways you can use diet and sleep management to safely and positively affect your moods and emotions.

Diet and Mood

Most of us realize that certain foods help us to feel better— ice cream and chocolate being just two examples. What most of us do not know is that *every meal dramatically influences our mood*. Not only does food change how we feel, but it does so rapidly. Brain chemistry and function can be influenced by a single meal. That is, in well-nourished individuals consuming normal amounts of food, short-term changes in the food consumed can rapidly affect brain function.

This means that you can combat depression and feelings of low self-esteem by changing the way you eat.

According to scientific research, carbohydrates stimulate the brain's production of a chemical neurotransmitter called serotonin. Serotonin creates feelings of well-being and inner peace; it calms anxiety, alleviates depression, and produces sounder sleep.

People who eat calming foods containing carbohydrates report feeling more relaxed, more focused, less stressed, less distracted after a meal. Behavioral tests that objectively rate performance prove that people tend to score better on tests that require concentration and focus after they eat a carbohydrate-rich meal. After people eat carbohydrates, feelings of stress and tension are eased and the ability to concentrate is enhanced. On the other hand, scientists have found that meals rich in animal protein cause a depletion of serotonin.

Because the McDougall Program for Maximum Weight Loss is so rich in carbohydrates, it is ideal for those who need to lose weight—and improve their moods. Increased serotonin also suppresses hunger, which of course reduces food cravings. The net effect of the McDougall diet is to encourage feelings of well-being, improve mood, sharpen concentration, and reduce appetite. All these factors make it easier to stay on the diet and to lose weight.

A Healthier Body Means a Healthier Mind

In a broad sense, improving health relieves depression. The pain, worry, and hopelessness that accompany illness can bring even the strongest people to their knees. Improved physical health will be reflected in improved mental health and emotional spirit. Improvement in general health should also mean less need for medications that cause depression, such as beta-blocker blood pressure pills and tranquilizers.

But there are other lifestyle and dietary measures you can take to relieve depression. Among the quickest are to increase exercise; stop drinking alcohol, which is a depression-inducing drug; stop drinking coffee, an anxiety-producing drug that can bring on depression during withdrawal; and, finally, reduce the number of hours you sleep.

Sleep Management for Mood Control

This next suggestion is for anyone who wants to try a natural way to improve mood and relieve depression. It's especially helpful for those who have not responded to medication for depression. The treatment: sleep management.

A growing body of research shows that too much sleep can cause a variety of mental disorders, including depression, in large numbers of people. Because sleep causes depression, it is referred to as "depressogenic" in the psychological literature. Wakefulness is antidepressogenic. Depressed patients, who are likely to respond to sleep deprivation, characteristically feel worse in the morning and gradually become freer of their symptoms as evening approaches, as the depressant effect of the previous night's sleep wears off through the wakeful hours of the day.

I have been recommending sleep management to my patients for years, with remarkable results. One of my patients, Max, is a seventy-year-old man who had recently retired. Suddenly Max had time on his hands, so he started getting ten hours of sleep each night. Like most of us, he thought this was a good idea. But in no time he realized that he had become terribly depressed. Max chalked up his depression to his retirement and all the well-known side effects retirement can have: loss of purpose; too much time available and too little to do; feelings of having been put out to pasture. One of Max's physicians prescribed Prozac, an antidepressant drug, but the medication made Max severely ill—so ill, in fact that he had to stop taking the drug. Max felt as if he had entered a world veiled in darkness. Even worse, he believed that the rest of his life would be spent in depression. He felt hopeless.

Max had been depressed for two years before he came to me. I immediately suggested that we get him on a sleep management program. I directed him to decrease the number of hours he slept each day from ten to seven, and then to six. Within two days of starting the program, Max's depression was gone. He felt great. And suddenly he had a wealth of creative ideas about what he could accomplish with all the time he had. Max has not been depressed since he began the sleep management program.

Recently, while I was doing my radio talk show, a woman called and explained that she suffered from long-term depression. I asked her how many hours a day she slept. Eight to ten hours a day was her answer. She told me she had been taught that the more sleep one got, the better one felt and looked— the old "beauty rest" wives' tale. I asked her to cut down to six or seven hours a day. A few weeks later, she called in to the radio show again and told me that her depression had been cured. The only day when she had experienced depression since she began the program, she said, was the day her husband forgot to set the alarm clock.

From earliest childhood, we have been taught that sleep is good for us—in fact, the more the better. The standard advice is that if we are to maintain health, we should get a minimum of eight hours each night. And indeed, such advice is reinforced by the refreshment derived from a good night's sleep and the associated relief from pain and worry we enjoy while we're asleep.

Young people need more sleep than adults. A newborn baby

may spend up to three-quarters of its day asleep, and children usually need eight to ten hours of sleep each night. Pregnancy temporarily increases the need for rest. So does illness.

However, in adulthood, eight hours a night is usually too much sleep for most people. Many of us actually feel and function best on five, six, or seven hours a night. Some people do well on less than five hours of sleep. As we age, sleep requirements diminish. Some elderly people, for example, can get all the sleep they need in three or four hours each night. Often insomnia occurs when you try to get more sleep than your body actually needs. In this case, the body is compensating for your enforced attempts at overresting it.

People who change to a high-carbohydrate diet also report less time spent sleeping, more restful sleep, and an increase in dream activity.

Sleep-Deprivation Therapy

A scientific review of sixty-one studies published between 1969 and 1990—studies that took place in thirteen countries and involved more than 1,700 patients—found that an average of 59 percent of patients showed a marked decrease in depressive symptoms the day after a night of sleep deprivation. Sixty-seven percent of people diagnosed with "endogenous depression"—or depression that has no apparent cause—responded positively to sleep deprivation. Sleep-deprivation therapy has also been helpful to patients suffering from depression related to other common situations, such as premenstrual syndrome.

Staying awake all night permits the washout of the depressant effects of the previous night's sleep. Usually, complete relief of depression is attained after a single sleepless night.

For many people, improvement of mood after sleep deprivation can last for several weeks. When the depression recurs, they merely restrict the number of hours they sleep again, which dissipates the depression. For some, a single full night's sleep is enough to cause a relapse of depression. Some patients are so sensitive to the depressing effects of sleep that they relapse even after a nap of two to fifteen minutes.

After a period of treatment with a carefully scheduled program, even many of these fragile people can control their depression.

Practical Sleep Management

The elevation of mood by controlling sleep is not limited to people who are severely depressed. Two studies reported improvement in people of "normal" mood who were deprived of sleep. Hence, manipulation of your sleeping habits has the potential to improve your mood, even if you do not perceive that you are depressed.

To gain the benefits of sleep deprivation, you needn't go completely without sleep. For many people, even partial deprivation is as effective as total deprivation in relieving depression. Studies have shown that this approach is more effective when a patient is awakened at 2 A.M. and kept awake until 10 P.M. than when the patient's bedtime is delayed. This pattern still allows for four hours of sleep per night, which is enough to relieve the fatigue expected from total loss of sleep. For many people, long-term relief of depression is accomplished with the use of partial sleep deprivation once every two to five days. This technique is simply used "as needed" to elevate mood and relieve depression.

In this way, sleep management can be tailored to meet the needs of the individual. You will determine the "right amount" of sleep for you by trial and error, and by closely observing your own response to sleep. In any case, you should experiment with your sleeping hours to achieve the right balance between fatigue and the benefits of fewer hours of sleep.

If you are depressed now, try cutting out one to two hours of sleep each night. You'll need a day or two to allow your body to adjust to the loss of sleep. But you may also expect an elevation of your mood after a couple of days. Add or subtract half an hour of sleep based on your mood and your fatigue.

The Triple Whammy

Diet, sleep management, and exercise all have a powerful effect on mood. Moreover, each enhances the effectiveness of the other. A high-carbohydrate diet combined with exercise increases the effectiveness of sleep management. Also, the correct amount of sleep will elevate your mood sufficiently to help you stay on a healthy diet and exercise program. All three are highly effective, cost-free, and nontoxic, and offer rapid results. Unfortunately, because such tools are hard to manipulate for profit, they are unlikely to get widespread attention or achieve much popularity.

Still, they are yours for the taking—free of charge and ready to change your life for the better today.

CHAPTER 12

Establishing a Healthy Way of Life

Now that you know the diet and exercise program and why it will work, you must confront the final obstacle to weight loss: yourself.

That sentence is going to deflate a lot of my readers, because down deep you blame yourself for your many failed attempts at weight loss, despite your heroic efforts. But that blame is both unfair and useless in your efforts to change. By now, you should realize that it wasn't possible for you to succeed on those other diets. All the sincere effort in the world isn't enough for you to overcome your hunger and your need for carbohydrates. Nor is it sufficient to overcome the effects of dietary fat. The McDougall Program for Maximum Weight Loss accommodates those needs while it causes you to lose weight.

One of the greatest obstacles to weight loss is not your inability to follow the program, but your lack of faith in yourself. Take, for example, the experience of Terry L. Murphy, a reporter for the *Niagara Gazette* in Niagara Falls, New York. In August 1990, Terry adopted my program so that she could write about it from firsthand experience. Here's part of Terry's report after being on the diet twelve days:

Like many people, I was hesitant to start a program that would eliminate a lot of what I thought I enjoyed. I worried McDougall's plan would preclude me from eating out with friends. I feared gaining weight, since I would be eating large quantities of starchy foods. I wondered if I could be as strict as McDougall wanted me to be. I worried that I would fail.

Well, I didn't fail. I ate out with friends. [In twelve days,] I lost five pounds. My cholesterol level dropped by 30 points (now it's 187). And I learned that I enjoyed feeling good a lot more than I enjoyed eating a hamburger.

If any of you have ever suffered from chronic digestive problems, you've learned to deal with the consequences of eating a meal: You eat, you feel ill. I wondered if McDougall's diet would rid my body of the stomach cramps that I had endured since childhood. It did. For the first few days I assumed it was just a fluke. After all, they didn't plague me every day. By the end of the first week, I was convinced of the connection. By the end of the twelfth day, I was confident that if I didn't want to suffer digestive problems ever again, I would have to make McDougall's diet a part of my lifestyle.

Fear of failing on any diet is as common as dieting itself. Anyone who considers adopting my program immediately wonders whether he or she has the discipline to stick to it. But you must take into consideration three important factors that will support you once you begin: (1) how good you will feel; (2) how the nutritional balance of the diet supports your sticking with it; and, not least, (3) how easily you will lose weight. These results make staying on the diet easier, because you experience the program's rewards. However, you cannot have the experience until you adopt the program and see for yourself.

Therefore, I have outlined the following simple steps to help you overcome your fear of failure. All these steps are designed to help you change. Once you have made a sincere effort at adopting the McDougall Program for Maximum Weight Loss, you'll recognize how easy and rewarding it is. But not until you begin to implement the program will you actually know that. So begin your new life. Confront your fears and resistance and change yourself for the better.

Here's how you can do it.

Step 1. Be Goal-Oriented

Establishing clear goals is the starting point for improved health. Follow these steps in establishing goals.

- Be specific. You need clear goals to know where you are going, how well you are progressing, and finally, when you have achieved your ambition.

Goals such as "I want to feel better" or "I want to look better" are too vague. Instead, decide that you want to lose thirty pounds in the next four months. You want to stop taking all three of your blood pressure pills and have a normal blood pressure. You want to walk five miles without chest pains. You want to wake up every morning without joint stiffness.

Be clear about all measurable goals, such as weight, waist measurement, dress size, blood pressure, and cholesterol level. This way, each time you show an improvement, you'll feel better about yourself; you'll have more faith in the program and yourself, and you'll realize that you will not be "forever fat" or "incurably ill." You'll also realize that you are capable of accomplishing what you set out to do.

- Put your goals in order. What are the things you want most to accomplish?
- Be realistic, but make goals challenging. You're not going to lose thirty pounds in a week unless a surgeon removes a watermelon-sized tumor from your belly. On the other hand, don't aim so low that your goal doesn't require you to change.
- Write down your goals and put them somewhere in your house where you will see them regularly to reinforce their place in your life.
- Think of all the reasons why you want to achieve each goal. For example: "I want to lose weight because I want to be more attractive to my spouse." Or "Looking better will make me more effective in my job." Or "Excess weight is a threat to my life."

These personal reasons will provide you with the motivation you need to overcome obstacles. Also, setting goals will help you overcome the tendency to do nothing about your health until it's too late.

To help you clarify your goals and adopt a timetable for their achievement, I have come up with the following form. Answer the questions and review the form and your answers frequently.

Identification of Health Goals

My short- and long-term goals for my appearance are:

- Lose weight: _____ pounds in _____ weeks; or _____ pounds in _____ months

- See the rippling of my muscles and outlines of my bones in _____ months.

- Keep myself trim and fit for:
  _____ three months.
  _____ six months.
  _____ one year.
  _____ the rest of my life.

- Bring the color back into my complexion in _____ months.

- Eliminate greasy skin in _____ week(s).

- Eliminate greasy hair in _____ week(s).

- Appear more graceful and agile in _____ months.

My short- and long-term goals for my health are:

- Lower my cholesterol by: _____ 25 mg/dl; _____ 50 mg/dl; _____ 100 mg/dl; _____ 150 mg/dl; or _____ to normal (below 150 mg/dl).

- Lower my triglycerides by: _____ 100 mg/dl; _____ 200 mg/dl; _____ 500 mg/dl; *or* _____ to normal (less than 200 mg/dl).

- Lower my blood pressure by: _____ 10/10 mmHg; _____ 15/15 mmHg; _____ 20/20 mmHg; *or* _____ to normal (110/70 mmHg or less).

- Lower my blood sugar: _____ 50 mg/dl; _____ 100 mg/dl; _____ 200 mg/dl; *or* _____ to normal (less than 115 mg/dl).

- Relieve my acid indigestion: _____ Some; _____ All.
- Relieve my constipation: _____ Some; _____ All.
- Relieve my postnasal drip and sinus: _____ Some; _____ All.
- Relieve my headaches: _____ Some; _____ All.
- Relieve my arthritis: _____ Some; _____ All.
- Feel energetic: _____ A little; _____ A lot.

- Reduce or eliminate medications:
  Blood pressure medications: _____ Some; _____ All.
  Diabetic pills: _____ Some; _____ All.
  Antacids: _____ Some; _____ All.
  Laxatives: _____ Some; _____ All.
  Painkillers: _____ Some; _____ All.
  Other medications (name):

  _____ : _____ Some; _____ All.

  _____ : _____ Some; _____ All.

  _____ : _____ Some; _____ All.

    in _____ days; _____ weeks; _____ months.

- Live to a healthy old age of: _____ 50; _____ 60; _____ 70; _____ 75; _____ 80; _____ 85; _____ 90; _____ 95; _____ 100.

My other short- and long-term goals are:

- _____ .
- _____ .
- _____ .
- _____ .

Here's another form to help you clarify all the reasons why you want to change and achieve your goals. Fill out the form and refer to it regularly.

Motivating Reasons to Change

The reasons I want to fulfill my goals are:

_____ I only live once and I want the most out of my life.

_____ I love my work and I will not be able to accomplish my ambitions without good health and my best appearance.

_____ I like to feel physically, mentally, and emotionally good about myself (I want to like myself again).

_____ I like the attentions I receive from others when I look good.

_____ I enjoy the physical freedom of bending over and tying my shoes.

_____ I enjoy walking, bicycling, swimming, and other physical activities and sports.

_____ I do not like the side effects of medications.

_____ I like the idea of being independent of drugs (drug-free).

_____ I do not enjoy pain (as common as indigestion and as horrible as the incisions from bypass surgery).

_____ I fear long suffering from cancer and other chronic diseases.

_____ I fear the treatments given for cancer, heart disease, arthritis, kidney failure, and other chronic diseases.

_____ I consider spending money on poor health foolish and wasteful.

_____ I dread being a burden on my family or friends.

_____ I fear dying prematurely.

My other motivating reasons for acomplishing my goals:

_____ .

_____ .

_____ .

_____ .

_____ .

_____ .

_____ .

Step 2. Acknowledge Your Willingness to Pay the Price

There is no such thing as a free lunch. How badly do you want your body to be trim? Well-established goals can help you determine the price you must pay to reach your goals. Then you must resolve in advance to pay that price.

When you want something badly enough, you will have the excitement, enthusiasm, energy, and endurance to achieve it. If you were dying in an intensive-care unit with tubes poking out of all your orifices, you would have the overpowering goal of staying alive, and you would resolve to pay whatever price was necessary. Unfortunately, in this critical situation your future is often beyond your control. Right now, happily, you have an opportunity; you're not condemned to obesity, and you're not hopelessly ill. You can lose the excess weight and regain your vitality.

To help you understand the price you are willing to pay for the achievement of your goals, I have composed the following form.

Paying The Price

Steps I must take to fulfill my goals:

- I will change my diet:

  Half-Hearted Approach:
  _____ Switch to low-fat dairy products.
  _____ Give up beef and pork for chicken and fish.
  _____ Skin my chicken.
  _____ Eat more vegetables.
  _____ Give up desserts.

  Serious Business:
  _____ Eat at home more often.
  _____ Avoid all oil like a poison.
  _____ Learn to prepare five new healthy meals now.
  _____ Try two new recipes a week.
  _____ Find two restaurants that serve healthful food.
  _____ Recruit two friends to follow the program with me.
  _____ Limit feasting to very special occasions.
  _____ Follow the most effective lifelong diet plan ever (The McDougall Program for Maximum Weight Loss).

- I will exercise:
  _____ I will walk, bicycle, swim, etc., _____ twice weekly; _____ every other day; _____ daily; _____ twice a day.
  _____ I will join an exercise class.
  _____ I will join a health club.

- I will confront my tobacco addiction: _____ Cut down; _____ Quit.
- I will confront my caffeine addiction: _____ Cut down; _____ Quit.
- I will confront my alcohol addiction (habit): _____ Cut down; _____ Quit.

- I will confront my illicit drug addiction (habit): _____ Cut down; _____ Quit.

- I will resolve psychological problems by:
  _____ Improving my diet and lifestyle.
  _____ Managing my sleep.
  _____ Keeping active.
  _____ Participating in hobbies and sports.
  _____ Changing employment.
  _____ Seeking marriage and family counseling.
  _____ Resolving conflicts with others.
  _____ Becoming active in my religious faith.
  _____ Seeking professional help.

Other activities:

_____ .

_____ .

_____ .

Step 3. Educate Yourself; Become an Expert

Every one of us has made mistakes because of simple ignorance. We ate certain foods because we didn't know they were bad for our health. Now we know better. We change by (first) becoming aware of the consequences of our mistakes, and (second) learning that there are alternatives. Then we begin to implement those alternatives, and soon we've developed a new way of living—a better way.

Take thirty minutes each day to learn more about health and nutrition. Look for new foods. Find new recipes. Think about your goals and the reasons you want to achieve them. Listen to audio- and videotapes and read books that promote healthful eating and living. The more you understand about health, the greater your chance of permanent success. The more you know, the better your opportunities will be to share your ideas with those around you.

Step 4. Visualize Yourself as Healthy

Picture yourself as slender, fit, and vital. Visualize that you do not take blood pressure medication, or have no chest pain, and that you enjoy robust good health. Perhaps you can remember a time when you weren't overweight and felt great.

Put this image in your mind often. The more you think of yourself as a healthy person, the more you will want to be that person and the harder you will work to achieve your goals.

Step 5. Make a Commitment: It's Magic

Not until you have fully committed yourself to a path can you actually travel along it. Every uncommitted act is doomed to fail from the outset. Failure to commit means that you are offering only a fraction of yourself to the endeavor, and even then your effort is undecided.

Commitment allows you to dedicate your entire being to the task at hand. You will be surprised at the way your environment responds to your commitment. Unexpected and incredibly supportive events occur. As the great mythologist Joseph Campbell said, follow your bliss and the universe miraculously supports your choices for a happier and healthier way of life. Therefore, give yourself fully to the task of making yourself healthy, happy, and beautiful. The goal is worth achieving, and you deserve that achievement.

Remember that you fulfill commitment by remaining focused on your intention and goals. Plan ahead. Have your house well stocked with foods used in the McDougall Program for Maximum Weight Loss. Pack your lunch for work or school. Call ahead to the kitchen that is serving your business banquet to order steamed vegetables without butter or cheese as your entree. If you're going to a friend's to eat, make sure that either you bring food or suitable food is provided for you. When appropriate, you can make suggestions as to what you like for dinner, or offer to contribute a dish.

Eat first when you're going to be confronted with rich foods.

It will enable you to resist temptation. Your control will be the envy of those around you.

Practice polite ways of declining foods, such as, "No thanks. Those scrambled eggs look delicious. But I'm under doctor's orders to avoid cholesterol." "I just had a big lunch, so I'll have to pass on those hamburgers."

Shop for food on a full stomach; your purchases will be guided more by your head than your old habits. Shopping with a list and a budget helps, especially when you consider the expense of red meat, dairy products, and processed and packaged foods.

Here's a form to help you with commitment.

I earnestly make this commitment:

I will expend all the effort necessary to accomplish my goals.

I will avoid fat-filled, rich foods.

I will exercise (type _____) _____ minutes a day.

If success is not easily accomplished, I will reexamine the principles of this program in light of my behavior, and try again.

If I fail initially I will consider the setback a learning experience, necessary for future success, and I will try again. I will reward myself for the smallest improvements, for they are all great accomplishments.

Signed: _____

Date: _____

DISCARDING EXCUSES

There are dozens of great excuses for avoiding proper diet and exercise. In case you are short on fresh ideas, here are some popular rationalizations.

I Like Being Fat

- I like being big; people respect me more.
- When I'm fat I don't have to deal with advances from the opposite sex.
- My spouse fell in love with me at this size and would leave me if I became thin.
- My spouse becomes jealous when I'm thin and attractive to other people.
- I lost weight once and people said I looked too thin. I couldn't take the pressure.
- People would think I was ill if I lost weight.
- I'd look like a starving refugee if I lived on what they ate, rice and potatoes.
- If I lost weight I'd have more wrinkles and would look ten years older.

I'm Not Worth the Trouble

- I'm too old to care about how I look.
- I'm not worth the trouble or deserving of a gorgeous body.
- I want to be irresistible, seductive, daring, mysterious, virtuous, modest, and thin; if I can't have it all, then I'll just stay fat.
- Obesity is my curse for being a horrible (or sinful) person.

It's Out of My Control

- My weight is inherited; big bones run in our family.
- My fat hips come from having babies.
- Everyone knows women have more trouble losing weight.
- Eating is my only pleasure.
- My life is too stressful right now for me to consider any changes in my diet.
- The life of a top executive is full of stresses that make me eat all the wrong things.

- In the world of business there are social obligations, with dinner and drinks, that I can't ignore.
- I'm too weak. I break down when I get hungry, angry, lonely, or tired.
- My doctor said I'm incurably fat; I have too many fat cells and too slow a metabolism.
- Even if I lose weight, I can't change my basic body shape anyway. Once a pear, always a pear (or once an apple, always an apple).
- Scientific research says I'm better off staying fat than gaining and losing weight.
- It will take months (or years) to lose all my weight.
- I've been on a hundred diets and I always regain my weight. In the short term I might see benefits, but nobody can stick to a diet.
- "Going on a diet" implies "going off" it.
- I'm angry with myself (or my spouse).

It's Too Difficult to Change

- I could never learn to like other foods.
- I don't like to cook and I don't want to learn how.
- It's too much work to shop, plan menus, and prepare meals.
- You just can't find foods that are low in calories.
- I don't have time to exercise.
- I eat out all the time. You can't find healthy, nonfattening foods in restaurants.
- My family will never eat that way. My spouse has to have meat, cheese, and fat to be happy.
- I don't want to do it all by myself.
- I don't want to be different. My friends would never put up with my special diet.
- Eating healthfully can be a burden on a full social calendar.
- I'm looking for the quick fix—drugs or surgery.
- Scientists are about to make a major breakthrough in obesity. I'll wait for the magic "cure."
- The pleasure of eating can make a lonely evening much more tolerable.
- Food means love, comfort, and safety—any change might mean I'd be worse off than I am already.

The Mother of All Excuses, and Its Solution

Let's face it, all these excuses boil down to one single excuse: We simply don't want to change. Change is scary. It takes us into the unknown. The unknown frightens us. Our current life may be filled with problems, but at least we know the problems we face. We're familiar with them. For the most part, we can cope with our current pains, failures, and disappointments. Deep down, we're secretly afraid that any new change will actually make our lives worse.

All of us resist growth to some extent. It's built in; I'm convinced of it. To paraphrase Tom Hanks's character in the movie *A League of Their Own,* if growth were easy, everybody would be doing it. But that's what makes it great.

In order to grow, we must overcome one aspect of our humanness that is not particularly pretty: the part of us that creates dark and negative pictures of the future. We keep ourselves from growing by imagining that life will get worse if we change. So we stay put, hunker down, stagnate, and pass our days dreaming of a better life without making any effort to create a better reality. You don't realize that some part of your brain is spinning out little scenarios of how much worse your future will be if you change. This keeps you from growing into a better and happier existence.

What I am about to tell you is so utterly simple and true that it may deceive you: Health feels better than sickness. You will be happier at your ideal weight than you are overweight. You will be proud of yourself. You'll have confidence. You'll feel so many good things that right now you cannot imagine and I cannot describe. But the net effect is that you'll like yourself a lot more. You'll look in the mirror and actually like what you see; you may even love what you see. You will have honored the person within yourself who longs to be healthy, beautiful, and free of all those burdens that overweight brings. Life will not be perfect, but it will be better.

And it's easy to accomplish. All you have to do is commit yourself to following the McDougall Program for Maximum Weight Loss. It works.

You do not have to be a gourmet cook to make your food delicious, either. Just follow the recipes and practice cooking the food. In a very short time, you will be preparing delicious, healthful, and weight-reducing meals. Day by day, you'll be making your best effort at creating better health. And day by day, you'll find yourself looking better, weighing less, and feeling more energy and confidence. It doesn't happen without effort. But that's what makes it great. You earn the right to be healthier, happier, more vital, beautiful, and alive. Enjoy it. You deserve to look and feel great.

Step 6. Ensure That Your Environment Supports Your Goals

Some people subscribe to the philosophy that if the cure doesn't hurt, it can't be working. When it comes to permanent changes in diet and lifestyle, the opposite philosophy is the best: The less painful the program, the more likely it is to succeed. Take steps to make your new life easier. Modify your daily behavior so that your surroundings work for you, not against you. Have the right pots, pans, and utensils to cook with; have the right spices, herbs, and seasonings to make your meals delicious; have your cookbooks handy and review them often to make your dishes lively and appealing.

Make sure you give yourself the time to shop for food and cook your meals. Change your life to support your health. Don't sacrifice your health for worthless conveniences.

Avoid temptation. Very few people could quit smoking without ridding their house of cigarettes. Alcoholics avoid bars to stop drinking. Protect yourself by protecting your environment. Decrease the time when you are exposed to rich foods to avoid testing your "willpower." One of the best ways to do this is to throw all the rich foods out of the house. Just as important is to replace harmful foods with those used in the McDougall Program for Maximum Weight Loss.

If many of your meals are eaten away from home, make the situations meet your needs. Go to restaurants that offer at least one delicious, nutritious item. Ask the waiter to remove the butter and olive oil from the table. Accept invitations to dinner from friends who eat and live healthfully. Bring healthful foods with you whenever possible.

Keep those people close who support your efforts and do not try to sabotage you. Ask family and friends to stop giving you boxes of candy and cakes as gifts. Instead suggest flowers, a card, or a fruit basket. Tell your mother that if she really loves you she'll feed you properly, forgoing her traditional beef stroganoff.

Step 7. Alter Your Coping Mechanisms

Instead of gorging on chocolate pie when you're hungry, angry, lonely, or tired, fill up on leftover Mexican Potato Salad or "Fried" Rice. Better yet, go for a walk; play your favorite sport; start working on an enjoyable project or hobby; visit a friend or go to a movie (and eat popcorn without butter). The best responses are those that involve physical activity, since they do double duty by reducing intake of fat calories and increasing calorie expenditure. If you must alleviate your frustration by eating, eat the right foods.

Step 8. Join a Support Group

Join a support group if you can. If there isn't one in your area, start one. Ideally, your support group will be following the same principles of good health—a group of McDougallers, or Pritikins, or followers of macrobiotic or natural hygiene will do. In Wheeling, West Virginia, there is a group of people who have McDougall potluck lunches every Tuesday afternoon. Even such organizations as Weight Watchers, TOPS (Take Off Pounds Sensibly), and OA (Overeaters Anonymous) may serve your needs for companionship and support, though the dietary education will not be what you're looking for.

You can start your own group by placing an ad in the newspaper that offers a potluck dinner for people interested in the McDougall Program; or run an ad offering to start a support group for those who want encouragement to lose weight and restore health. From there, things can take off rapidly.

Meanwhile, find new friends who are also involved in healthful approaches to life by frequenting health-food stores and restaurants or by attending lectures.

Groups can be as small as two. The chance of success is increased tremendously if your spouse or partner also follows a healthful diet and exercise program. If your partner rejects your efforts to regain your health, he or she should consider what it would feel like to be sleeping next to an empty place at night, instead of you. Encourage your present friends to be active so that you can continue to enjoy recreation with them.

Step 9. Reward Yourself

When you make a good choice, pat yourself on the back or give yourself a gold star on your forehead. You deserve rewards along the way. Buy yourself a new dress or a new set of golf clubs with all the money you're saving by giving up your high-fat diet or liquid-protein regimen. Ask yourself what you want for yourself, your house, or some other special purpose, and make that a reward for your hard work and accomplishment. You'll be able to afford a lot of things with the savings you accumulate from brown-bagging your lunch instead of eating out, and from discarding those expensive antacids and other medications, which you'll be able to give up soon after adopting the McDougall Program for Maximum Weight Loss.

Step 10. Keep It Simple

You may be thinking that adopting my program will take a lot of work. You may be saying that you don't want to make life any more complicated than it is right now. But you do not realize how complicated it already is, and how simple you can make it by improving your health. You may currently be burning a piece of flesh on two sides and calling it a convenient dinner, but it takes no more time to steam vegetables, cook a grain, microwave or boil potatoes and cover them with barbecue sauce, and boil some frozen broccoli. If, on the other hand, you like to cook, you can make any of the recipes in this or many of those in the other McDougall books.

Most people enjoy a small variety of foods regardless of the kind of diet they're on or the effort they make to prepare their meals. Usually they have the same thing for breakfast, one or two of the same things for lunch, and a half dozen favorites for dinner. These foods are merely rotated through the month. It's the same at restaurants; people order the same favorite meal from the menu every time they go out.

It can be that easy on the McDougall Program for Maximum Weight Loss. You can develop a repertoire of fewer than a dozen recipes that are both enjoyable and quick. Soon you will have learned the ingredients you must have on hand and the routine for cooking your meals.

Health Is Everything (If You Lose It)

Fear can be a great motivator. Perhaps deep down you're afraid of where your health is going, or what kind of crisis may be in the offing if you persist in your current way of life. Even though your body is very forgiving of your mistreatment, there is a limit to the abuse it can take. I hope this chapter on motivation—with all the positive incentives that are implicit in adopting this program—will be enough to help you make the changes that are necessary. But if it is not, consider the current direction of your life. I hope these thoughts alone will motivate you to change before disaster strikes.

All of you reading this book have the advantage of knowing the most effective solutions for your problems with health and appearance—the McDougall Program for Maximum Weight Loss. Serious health problems can become motivators for those of us who can see past our false sense of invincibility.

CHAPTER 13

Beauty and Health

Attractiveness—even beauty—begins with health. Health is the underlying radiance that glows from beneath the skin. Health imbues every aspect of your physical and psychological being. It inspires your every movement; it provides balance to your emotions; it makes your mind sharp while giving you greater tolerance and understanding of others. The signs of health are recognized by everyone: glowing, clean skin, a firm body moving with agility and grace. People who are unhealthy tend to have short tempers, greater emotional ups and downs, wide swings in energy, and—obviously—an array of unpleasant physical symptoms. Health is the ultimate integrator, unifying the most tangible physical aspects of our being with the loftiest and most spiritual. Health is so much more than body weight, but it does provide the basis for normal weight. Even more, health is the foundation of beauty.

We all recognize a healthy appearance when we see it, and no amount of makeup will camouflage the look of poor health.

Youth is associated with an attractive appearance, largely because young people are usually still healthy. As people age, they commonly lose their health, and this decay is reflected in a loss of attractiveness. But it doesn't have to be so. You can't stop the passage of years, but you can moderate the toll time takes on you and the way you look. To look your best during every decade of life, you must take advantage of the benefits of eating and living well.

Even after years of abuse, people regain their health and attractiveness when they change their diet and lifestyle. I see the dramatic changes in less than two weeks at my clinic at St. Helena Hospital; in twelve days, people become healthier and seem to grow younger. The change is evident to their fellow patients and the clinic staff, but is particularly striking to family who have not seen them for twelve days.

Beautiful Teeth, Skin, and Hair, and a Healthy Smile

Sugar is widely known as a cause of tooth decay. However, few people recognize that other substances contribute to the health and longevity of your teeth and gums. Among the most important of these are vitamins, minerals, fiber, and protein. A diet high in animal protein depletes calcium and causes the loss of the bones that hold the teeth. A combination of a healthy diet and excellent dental hygiene, including flossing, frequent brushing, and regular visits to the dental hygienist, can reverse serious gum disease—and in many cases avoid surgery.

In the Pink

Red blood cells, shaped like tiny doughnuts, carry oxygen from your lungs to tissue cells throughout your body. These red cells, which are about 7.5 microns (millionths of a meter) in diameter, are capable of fitting into tiny blood vessels, called capillaries, that are only 3.5 microns in diameter. Like so many circus clowns that can climb into a Volkswagen, these red blood cells are highly flexible; they can bend in half in order to fit into the smallest of your body's capillaries so that no cell in your body is deprived of oxygen.

However, within minutes of consuming the standard American high-fat meal, tiny balls of fat pour into the bloodstream and coat individual red cells, causing them to stick together in clumps. When fat-coated, the red blood cells naturally become rigid and incapable of bending in half. Once they adhere to one another, these clumps of cells turn your circulation into sludge. In the smaller bottlenecks of your vessels, that sludge can literally cause your blood to stand still. The results are about a 20 percent drop in oxygen content of the blood and the suffocation of many of the body cells that are deprived of oxygen from these clumped red blood cells. This causes organs and tissues to function at less than optimal levels so that general health is affected.

In addition, the sludging of the blood changes the color of the skin. Blood cells become red when they receive oxygen from the lungs. After they deliver their oxygen load to the tissues, they receive carbon dioxide and then turn blue. With the circulation slowed by all that fat, a large amount of "blue" blood, deficient in oxygen, is present in the vessels, and is seen as a blue or gray tint in the skin. This is an all-too-common condition among light-skinned Caucasians, especially among the elderly, who often suffer from poor circulation as well as from heart and lung diseases. But poor circulation affects the skin of all races; healthy skin, no matter what its color, relies primarily on optimal circulation.

Within hours of removing fats and oils from the diet, circulation improves and the blue-gray tinge is replaced by a pink glow—a "rosy" complexion. The casual observer may overlook the color change, simply noticing that the person looks healthier. The actual color changes will be less evident in darker-skinned people, but the radiance that comes with enriched circulation will still be unmistakable.

Oily Skin and Hair

The skin, with its seemingly endless number of pores, is one of the body's major eliminative organs. The body attempts to eliminate excess fats, oils, and other toxins that we consume in our diets through the pores of our skin. Therefore, as a general rule, the better the diet the healthier the skin.

Specifically, excess oils and fats in our food are carried by the blood to the skin's surface, where the body attempts to rid itself of this burden to health via the pores. The more fats you consume, the oilier your skin and hair will be; however, even small amounts of fats in your diet may be noticeable and troublesome. The fat content of your diet will be reflected in your skin condition within hours of eating. When you reduce fatty and oily foods, you will see dramatic changes in the health of your skin. Even people who may think they have inherited tendencies to oily skin will see improvement in their skin condition when they change their diet. (Most "inheritance" is behavior learned from parents.)

Washing with soaps and shampooing once, twice, or more often every day are a losing battle for most oily-skinned people, because they cannot keep up with the constant outpouring of oil onto the skin and scalp. Fortunately, a very-low-fat diet such as the McDougall Program for Maximum Weight Loss will noticeably reduce surface oils in one to four days for almost everyone. (A few people will improve but will still have oily skin after the change in diet because large amounts of fat are being released from their own body fat. As weight loss stabilizes, these people almost always experience relief of oily skin.)

Occasionally people will complain of dry skin when following a diet very low in fat. They may even wonder whether they should increase the amount of fat in their diet to correct this condition. The answer is no. The healthiest response is for them to oil their skin from the outside rather than the inside, using a commercial moisturizing cream. A small amount of oil is absorbed from the skin into the body, but this is inconsequential.

A Clear, Clean Complexion

Eighty-five percent of all teenagers have acne at some time, and for many people skin trouble continues into adult life. Certainly the hormone surges that accompany puberty are related to increased skin oil (called sebum) and therefore contribute to acne. Nevertheless, acne is a preventable disease, not a normal condition. Fats from your fork and spoon are the most controllable cause of acne. On the skin's surface, bacteria feed on these fats and divide them into free fatty acids that irritate the skin and cause inflammation and infection. The results are pus-filled pimples.

People with acne who adopt a low-fat diet can improve the condition and reduce the amount of sebum their skin cells secrete. Once the oiliness of the skin is decreased, the pimples vanish. However, the threshold of tolerance for fats and oils is very small: One pepperoni pizza can mean a crop of pimples on your face that will last a week.

Oils and fats collect in large pores in the skin's surface, producing unattractive blackheads and whiteheads. These can be removed with an instrument, but they continue to recur as long as the fats continue to pour out through the skin and collect in the pores.

No Longer Puffy and Swollen

In the morning you may peer through puffy slits in your face. This puffiness comes from an accumulation of fluid caused by gravity while you are lying asleep. When you rise, gravity moves the fluids to your legs and feet.

The fluids that puff up the tissues underlying your skin are the direct result of the components of the foods you choose. Salt draws fluids into the tissues. Fats in the bloodstream slow circulation and cause bottlenecks. These areas of trapped blood cause fluids to escape the vessels and enter the tissues; the consequence is swelling. Fat also causes hormonal imbalances that further encourage swelling (edema).

However, a low-fat, low-sodium, high-carbohydrate diet improves circulation and flushes edema from the body. Fluid loss may be as much as a pound a day in people with severe edema—without the use of diuretics. Not only are the salt and fat reduced, but the carbohydrates in a healthful diet provide fuel for the cellular pumps that move salt and fluid out of tissues. Carbohydrates also provide energy for the kidney cells that eliminate this unwanted fluid from the body.

Resolving Rashes and Skin Diseases

As with other skin problems, unsightly skin diseases and rashes can be relieved by a change in diet. Eczema, for example, is often caused by dairy products and eggs. Some skin diseases, such as dermatitis herpetiformis, are caused by the gluten found in troublesome amounts in wheat, barley, and rye. Skin diseases are sometimes symptoms of more serious systemic diseases, such as lupus erythematosus and the deforming skin lesions of psoriasis. Both of these diseases are found commonly only among people who eat the rich Western diet. Many people are relieved of both the underlying conditions and the skin lesions they cause by changing to a low-fat diet free of animal products.

Hair in All the Right Places

Imbalances in the sex hormones of women can prevent ovulation and cause infertility, excessive hair growth, and acne. Often these symptoms also accompany ovarian cysts (otherwise known as polycystic ovaries). This is not an uncommon problem. In a recent study, 23 percent of women were found to have polycystic ovaries; of these, 76 percent had irregular menstrual periods and/or excess body hair. A change to a low-fat diet lowers levels of reproductive hormones and decreases hair growth and acne. As weight is reduced, cysts in the ovaries also disappear.

In men, the tendency toward male-pattern baldness is passed on genetically, but its development is not inevitable, even for men who have the "balding" gene. The loss of hair is the result of increased activity of sebaceous glands in the scalp, caused by overstimulation of these glands by the male hormone testosterone. In numerous populations, a correlation has been observed between increased levels of animal fats and higher levels of sebaceous-gland activity in the scalps of men. This condition is also associated with increased incidence of male-pattern baldness. Following a low-fat diet reduces male hormones and thereby prevents baldness in susceptible men. Once hair is lost, regrowth is difficult, but some doctors claim this is possible for some men with the aid of a low-fat diet and/or medications that reduce sebaceous-gland activity.

Strong Muscles and Straight Bones

Few things convey youth and vitality more than healthy muscle. But muscle is often the very tissue lost with "portion-controlled" semistarvation diets. Once you go off such a diet, the weight you regain is largely fat. This loss-gain cycle is repeated with each attempt to lose weight. The result is a body of the same predieting weight, with much more fat and much less muscle than before the dieting was started.

Muscle is not lost on the McDougall Program for Maximum Weight Loss because there is plenty of fuel for the body to use in the form of carbohydrate; there is no need to burn muscle fuel. Add a little exercise to the program and you'll gain muscle tone and muscle mass as you lose weight.

Pleasant Body Odor

We Americans are obsessed with body odor. We made the deodorant industry part of the *Fortune* 500. And we owe it all to our unhealthful way of eating.

Most foods and spices contain aromatic substances that affect the odors of our armpits, breath, urine, and stool. We fail to notice many odors simply because they have become so familiar. This occurs especially with odors in our homes and the places where we work. We simply stop noticing many smells until we enter a new environment. Often we fail to appreciate the effects of foods on the body odors of others because they eat the same foods we do. This is especially true of those who live together; even if they eat lots of garlic, onions, and spices, nobody notices.

You begin to appreciate the effects of food on body smells when you interact with people who eat differently. For example, authors writing about their experiences with traditional Eskimos often describe their fishy body odor. The spices of Asian,

Indian, Italian, Mexican, and other ethnic foods are carried on people's bodies. I first noticed the effects of food on body odor when I was a sugar plantation doctor taking care of vegetarian hippies who bathed infrequently. They smelled strongly of fruits and vegetables.

If food contributes so much to the odor of people, you may wonder what people smell like who eat products from cows, pigs, and chickens. In truth, the foulest odors come from putrefaction of animal products in the large intestine. There bacteria act on beef, poultry, eggs, and dairy products to produce malodorous gases that are passed with the flatus. These gases are also absorbed through the intestinal wall and into the bloodstream, which circulates them to the skin and lungs, where they are released as offensive body odors and bad breath. During the Vietnam and Korean wars, Asian soldiers claimed they could recognize the smell of decaying meat when downwind of American troops.

I will always remember one woman whose husband, a vegetarian, threatened divorce because of her body's unpleasant odor. Removal of meat, poultry, and dairy products from her diet saved their marriage. Several of my patients have complained about sour foot odors, which they say are relieved by eliminating dairy products.

As the Madison Avenue hucksters know, the body's fragrances are important catalysts of sexual attraction. Scientists have demonstrated the intimate connection of the nerve fibers of the olfactory lobes (our smell mechanism in the brain) and the hippocampus, the emotional center of the brain where our sexual drive originates. But it was never better put than by Napoleon, who wrote from the battlefield to Josephine: "Be home in three days. Don't wash."

The Sexual Male—Avoiding Impotence

As a plantation doctor living on the island of Hawaii nearly twenty years ago, I was struck by the reproductive abilities of many elderly male patients. After retirement from plantation work, some of the men would return to their native Philippines to find young brides. Daily I would be visited in my medical office by a family consisting of several young children, a wife in her twenties, and an older but very physically fit man. These sixty- and seventy-year-old men were not only fully functional—which is to say, reproductive—but highly optimistic. They planned to see their young children grow into adults, and usually managed to realize this goal. The reason for their remarkable health was their diet of rice and vegetables. Unfortunately, their offspring adopted the American diet rich in artery-damaging cholesterol and fat and became obese, sick, and impotent.

More frightening for many men than the loss of their life through a heart attack is the loss of their sexual and reproductive function through impotence. Impotence is the consistent inability to achieve or sustain an erection sufficient for sexual intercourse. This problem is different from other sexual problems that involve libido, ejaculation, and orgasm. In the United States approximately 10 million men are impotent.

The incidence of impotence increases with age: At forty years old, approximately 2 percent of men are affected; by age sixty-five, 25 percent of men cannot achieve a satisfactory erection.

The penis is made up largely of three bundles of spongy material, honeycombed with blood vessels. When filled to capacity with blood, the organ stands erect. This is accomplished by increasing the flow of blood into the penis while decreasing the outflow. The message to alter the blood flow and generate an erection can come from local sensory stimulation and from psychogenic stimulation in the brain (erotic thoughts, touches, sights, sounds, aromas, and tastes). The penis becomes flaccid when the amount of blood flowing into the organ decreases and the blood leaving increases.

Until recently it was thought that more than 95 percent of the time this problem was all in the man's head—psychogenic impotence. Performance anxiety and other fears surrounding the sex act are common among men, but this could not account for the insidious loss of function experienced by so many men as they aged.

Doctors now realize that most problems of impotence are not psychogenic, but have a physical cause, primarily diet. There are several common ways the rich American diet causes failure to achieve an adequate erection. By far the most common is hardening of the arteries (atherosclerosis) to the penis caused by a high-fat, high-cholesterol diet. This same underlying disease causes cholesterol plaques to form in the arteries leading to the heart and brain, and thereby causes heart attacks and strokes. Such blockage of blood vessels may account for as much as 80 percent of the impotence suffered by men in our society.

There are more erection-killing effects of diet. Excess dietary fat elevates levels of a hormone produced in the pituitary gland, called prolactin, which reduces the production and activity of male hormones. As many as 19 percent of men with impotence may have elevated levels of prolactin. Elevated levels of prolactin may also be caused by medications, such as antacids (cimetidine) and some blood pressure pills (methyldopa). These medications are used to treat diseases caused by the American diet.

Many other medications used to treat dietary diseases cause impotence. These include antihypertensive pills (for high blood pressure), antidepressants, tranquilizers, antiandrogens (which block male hormone activity), and anticholinergics (which block the parasympathetic nervous system). In one large study, sexually related side effects caused 8.3 percent of males to discontinue taking blood pressure pills.

Alcohol is probably the drug that most commonly causes both temporary and permanent sexual dysfunction. The high-fat American diet also causes prostate disease, including benign prostatic hypertrophy and prostate cancer. Both can lead to surgery and drug therapies that can have a profound effect on ability to perform sexually.

Sexual performance is intimately tied to personal appearance and physical fitness. If you can't bend over to tie your shoes, how do you expect your body to perform in this other important area? Some men are so ill that gathering the energy to make it through the day is all they can manage; concern for sustaining an erection is hardly a priority. Many men tell me that after attending my program at St. Helena Hospital, their sexual appetite and performance have returned. They feel and perform as if they were twenty years younger.

Sometimes a man's physical restoration stems both from improved health and from the elimination of medication. This is especially true for men who take medication for high blood pressure, which often has a debilitating effect on sexual performance.

Roy C. Weaver, a fifty-nine-year-old engineer from Reno, came to the McDougall Program for Maximum Weight Loss and lost forty pounds.

"I heard Dr. McDougall speak on KOH Radio in Reno, Nevada," Roy said. He heard my show after he had had coronary artery bypass surgery and was on an assortment of drugs for high blood pressure, adult-onset diabetes, and angina pectoris (pain in the chest caused by an insufficient supply of blood and oxygen to the heart). At the time of this writing, thirteen months after starting the program, Roy had lost nearly fifty pounds.

"It took me three months to change my way of eating, after I had bypass surgery," Roy said. "I lost the weight in six months, and have kept it off (while continuing to lose). I can eat twice as much food, and still lose weight. I am not hungry and have had none of that yo-yo syndrome. I have referred this plan to a minimum of twenty people, and the program saved my life."

Roy added, "I am into biking, and walking for about thirty minutes a day three to four times a week."

Other benefits: "I have a better complexion, with more vigor, have stopped the Lopressor and Micronase [high blood pressure and diabetes drugs, respectively]. I'm taking no medication of any kind now. All my vital signs have moved toward normal or have stabilized."

As for other programs, Roy said he tried "every kind known to man; success with none."

Roy is not the only person in his family who has benefited from the program: His wife, Virginia, has lost twenty-five pounds.

The Sexual Female

As with men, diet plays a fundamental role in the health of female sexuality and reproduction. And, of course, a woman's sexual and reproductive health have profound effects on her sense of her attractiveness, and ultimately on her appearance.

The standard American diet increases estrogen levels 50 percent above normal in many women. The breasts and uterus are highly sensitive to hormonal balance in all women. Overstimulation of the breast tissue by hormones leads to fibrocystic breast disease, characterized by painful cystic breast lumps. Almost all women have some tenderness before their menstrual periods; 50 percent of women are troubled by these symptoms, and 8 percent find their breasts so tender that the pain interferes with their normal daily activities. Continued overstimulation of the breasts by hormones leads to breast cancer for one in nine women. Deforming surgery—and/or high-dose radiation—often follows a diagnosis of breast cancer (and surgery sometimes follows a diagnosis of severe fibrocystic disease).

Overstimulation of the uterus by excess female hormones caused by the American diet leads to heavy, painful menstrual periods. After years of this excess stimulation, a condition of very heavy bleeding, called abnormal uterine bleeding, can develop. Hysterectomy is the common remedy. The other prevailing reason for hysterectomy is fibroids of the uterus caused by overstimulation of the uterine muscles by female hormones from the diet. Uterine cancer is another side effect of this high-fat eating, and hysterectomies are the unfortunate consequence. Many women feel a loss after such operations, which can lead to depression and decrease in sexual interest. They feel that "something important is missing"; in fact, something is missing because the uterus also produces lubricating fluids important for normal sexual intercourse.

Emotional disturbances related to cyclic hormones of women are collectively called premenstrual syndrome (PMS). PMS is characterized by tension, irritability, depression, anxiety, mood swings, sleep disturbances, abdominal bloating, edema, breast tenderness, and a craving for carbohydrate-rich foods. The typical craving for carbohydrates is an effort to help relieve the emotional disturbances of PMS by increasing the neurotransmitter serotonin, which relieves the symptoms and brings feelings of well-being.

Sheila Gill of Montara, California, and Dorothy Jones of Talmage, California, are two of many who can testify that the

McDougall Program for Maximum Weight Loss can result in more than just a slimmer figure.

Sheila Gill, forty-one years old, never could shake the additional weight she gained after her daughter was born. When she reached 140 pounds—the heaviest she'd ever been—she started searching for a program that would help her lose the weight. But Sheila had an additional incentive to be strict with her diet.

"I was diagnosed with 'early breast cancer' in 1989, and was told that the treatment of choice was a simple mastectomy," she said. "After a great deal of research and a hunch that such a procedure would weaken my entire body, and after consulting with Dr. McDougall, I decided to choose diet and lifestyle as my prescription for health and well-being. I had a lumpectomy only. So far it seems to be working. I feel great! I lost thirty pounds and now weigh 110 pounds at five feet, six inches tall. I am healthier overall. And since my diagnosis of breast cancer, which I realize is caused by fat, I've become much stricter. My body is less tolerant of abuse at my age."

Trial and error have proven to Sheila that the McDougall diet makes her feel the best. "I tried many diet plans, including Weight Watchers. They invariably recommended specific foods at specific times, with animal protein eaten in excess. Any high-protein, high-fat diet caused extreme tiredness and made me want sugar to raise my energy."

Like Sheila, seventy-year-old Dorothy Jones changed her way of eating in the face of a life crisis: She was diagnosed with colon cancer. "I started with the twelve-day program at St. Helena Hospital, and just continued," Dorothy said. "I eat more now than I used to; I don't have to sacrifice, or feel cheated, and there are no more confusing decisions on what to eat. In two months I lost all the weight that I wanted to—which was twenty-three pounds.

"I now have healthier hair, my eyes are clearer, I have a nicely shaped body, and my skin has cleared. I feel good about how I look and have taken more interest in clothes. I am full of energy. I wake up early, and have lots of reserve for the full day, even into the evening. I have the energy I had as a young woman. I know that I am treating my body the best that I can and I hope this has a favorable impact on my cancer. I get a good night's sleep now with a full but not loaded stomach. I have good digestion with regular and easy bowel movements. This way of eating is also good for the environment, economical, easy, and convenient; and it's fun!"

Dorothy's exercise program consists of "Nautilus Gentle Stretch for half an hour daily, and then golf, garden, and taking care of a large home." Clearly, her diet has dramatically improved the quality of her life, besides giving her a sense of control, vitality, and all the signs of health.

Lifelong Health

The normal human life span should be, on average, eighty-five years. As an individual with free will, armed with education, you have the chance to make the best of each of those years. If you haven't eaten the best diet or lived a healthy lifestyle, now is the time to start. The body is very forgiving and has a tremendous ability to recuperate. You will be surprised and pleased by the results you experience on the McDougall Program for Maximum Weight Loss. Don't waste another minute.

CHAPTER 14

Eating Out, the McDougall Way

Many people live on the run. They have neither the time nor the inclination to do much cooking at home. Following the McDougall Program for Maximum Weight Loss while eating out is simply a matter of finding a few places that serve the foods you like. People are creatures of habit—they order the same items from the menu time after time. One or two restaurants with healthful selections can keep you going for weeks or months. Low-fat vegetable dishes are so much in demand these days that almost every restaurant chef has learned to prepare a few items. You must be willing to ask questions, and be specific about the ingredients you want and don't want in your meal. Here is a guide to eating out—the McDougall way.

Restaurant Flavorings

Salad dressings are almost always laden with oils and/or dairy products, which makes the vast majority of them unacceptable. But just about any restaurant will provide you with a wedge of lemon or a dash of vinegar for your salad. Salt and black pepper are present on every table. Most of you can use these ingredients, sparingly, without adverse results. The catsup most restaurants serve is likely to have lots of sugar in it, and possibly too much salt, but at least it has no fat, so it may be acceptable if you use it sparingly.

Many restaurants are offering soy sauce these days, but some soy sauces contain monosodium glutamate (MSG). Not only is this ingredient high in sodium, but some people react adversely to the glutamate. Read the label on the bottle or ask what the soy sauce contains before using it.

You can bring along items from home to spice up your restaurant meals, such as low-fat, low-salt salad dressings, lemon juice, vinegar, tomato catsup, horseradish, Tabasco, Louisiana hot sauce, soy sauce, or any other condiments acceptable to your individual health plan. Many barbecue sauces packaged in jars have no oil but do contain a little sugar and salt. They may be acceptable.

Beverages

Order water—it's the ideal beverage. Nothing quenches thirst better or serves you more faithfully. For a little more sparkle, order seltzer or soda water (preferably without sodium). Noncaffeinated (herbal) teas are available in most restaurants or can be brought from home in individual packets. Every restaurant can supply you with hot water. A slice of lemon or lime can be added to any of the above for an additional fresh taste.

Practical Breakfast Suggestions

Hot cereals: Order oatmeal without butter, cream, or milk. If necessary, add sweeteners such as sugar, honey, maple syrup, or an artificial sweetener. One teaspoon (sixteen calories) of sugar on the surface of your cereal should be your limit. You may want to add a small amount of apple juice, orange juice, or other sweet juice instead. Because of their larger particle size, cooked whole grains are preferable to processed grain cereals such as cream of wheat and polenta (cooked cornmeal). Cooked whole-grain rice may be an option at some restaurants.

Cold cereals: Choose among the list of boxed cold cereals provided in "A Shopping List: McDougall-Okayed Packaged and Canned Products" in Chapter 15. Top with hot water or cold apple or orange juice, or bring along low-fat rice milk.

If no acceptable cold whole-grain cereals are available, you may decide to eat the next best choice, such as Shredded Wheat, NutriGrain cold cereals, Grape-Nuts, or Skinner's raisin bran. As a last resort, choose one of the more refined selections—one without added oils or dairy.

Fruits: Everywhere you eat you will find a selection of fruits. You will be limiting your daily intake to two a day.

Hash brown and home-fried potatoes: Home-fried potatoes are cooked white potatoes, cut in about one-inch chunks. Hash browns are grated boiled potatoes, often frozen in rectangular cubes. Ask whether you can get either of these cooked in a little water or on a dry skillet instead of in oil. Both home fries and hash browns turn nicely brown even without oil. If you can find nothing for breakfast that fits the McDougall Program for Maximum Weight Loss, choose foods that would fit the original McDougall Program, such as whole-wheat toast without butter (you may add a little jelly), bagels, pancakes, or waffles (all made with the right ingredients, of course).

Practical Lunch Suggestions

Baked potatoes: At less than 150 (mostly carbohydrate) calories each, you can afford to eat one, two, or more large potatoes. They're best eaten plain, or with some chives, onions, vegetable seasonings, lemon juice, and/or vinegar. You can also dust them with a light shake of table salt, soy sauce (without MSG), or Tabasco. Or if you prefer, bring along a spice bottle of your favorite blended seasonings, or an acceptable salad dressing, barbecue sauce, or Louisiana hot sauce. As a variation, break the potatoes with a fork into small pieces and mix thoroughly with your choice of spices, sauce, and/or dressing. You can top potatoes with an acceptable salad, soup, or sauce found in more health-conscious restaurants.

Salad bars: The popularity of salad bars has made them a fixture in fast-food establishments, supermarkets, and good restaurants. Not every ingredient on display is for you—too many are laced with gobs of oil, salt, and mayonnaise. Look closely and you'll be able to identify the vegetables covered with sauces and shining with oil. Use lemon juice, vinegar, or your own bottled low-fat, low-sodium dressing over the vegetables you collect. Sprinkle some no-salt seasoning blend over your salad. Most salad bars allow "all you can eat," so don't hesitate to take seconds.

Vegetable soups: More restaurants are serving what their health-conscience customers demand, such as excellent oil-free vegetable soup. Check the ingredients. They should be only vegetables, spices, and a little salt.

Fast meals from supermarkets: You can find assorted raw vegetables to serve as a snack or a lunch. Top with various acceptable dressings or condiments. (See Chapter 15, under "A Shopping List: McDougall-Okayed Packaged and Canned Products," for some suggestions.) Add a few rice cakes at thirty-five calories each. Acceptable packaged vegetable soups can be served up with the addition of hot water. (Again, you will find a list of acceptable soups in Chapter 15.)

A salsa-and-vegetable medley can be turned out in under two minutes. Get low-sodium, water-packed canned (or bottled) kidney beans, garbanzo, or other beans; acceptable salsa or salad dressing; a head of lettuce, and a few tomatoes, onions, and sprouts. Drain and mash the beans and top with chopped vegetables and salsa or salad dressing. You can heat all of this in a microwave oven if you like, but it's tasty enough to eat at room temperature or cold. As a variation, you might try Indian, Chinese, or Indonesian seasoning sauces. But be sure to check the ingredients.

If you cannot find foods that fit the McDougall Program for Maximum Weight Loss, choose foods that fit the original McDougall Program, such as a sandwich made with whole-grain bread (no oil, no dairy), lettuce, bean sprouts, tomatoes, onions, green peppers, and any other low-fat vegetables.

Buy a round of whole pita bread and a fruit or two. If that's too simple, fill the pita bread with lettuce, tomato, sprouts, and onions. Add some drained and mashed low-sodium, water-packed canned (or bottled) pinto beans or other beans and you'll have a delicious, hearty sandwich. Try filling a corn or whole-wheat tortilla with water-packed beans, lettuce, tomatoes, onions, sprouts, and your favorite salsa. The more vegetables you use, the more you are emphasizing the principles of the McDougall Program for Maximum Weight Loss.

Practical Dinner Suggestions

Seasoned steamed vegetables: Call several of the better restaurants in your area and ask whether they serve a steamed vegetable platter, and whether they will prepare yours without butter and cheese. The more expensive and fancier restaurants usually have a vegetable dish on the menu at a reasonable price. Generally the chef will add a special blend of spices and herbs to the dish before it reaches your table. If you think more zest is needed, sprinkle the vegetables with lemon juice, vinegar, or a low-fat salad dressing or favorite seasoning blend. If, after that, you're still hungry, order another serving. Be sure to have enough starchy vegetables with your order to satisfy your appetite.

Steakhouse choices: Steakhouses usually have great salad bars and baked potatoes. Bring along your own low-fat salad dressings or ask for vinegar and/or lemon juice. You can also order a platter of steamed vegetables on the side.

Mexican foods: Most Mexican foods are full of lard! But by telephoning ahead you can find a Mexican restaurant that does not use lard or vegetable oil in its beans, or at least one whose chef is willing to make your beans without either. Look for a place that serves whole beans rather than mashed beans, which are usually mixed with some type of fat. Order a plate of beans and rice with steamed vegetables on the side. At the very least, they'll be willing to serve you a side of lettuce and tomatoes as a salad. Any of these items can be topped with oil-free salsa served at the table.

As a variation from the stricter McDougall Program for Maximum Weight Loss, you might choose a flat tortilla, which is permitted on the original McDougall Program. Using low-fat beans, the chef can make you a bean tostada on a soft cornmeal shell (just cornmeal and lime, not fried). Or the chef can make a bean burrito from a soft whole-wheat tortilla shell. (More than likely the burrito shell will contain refined flour and a little oil, so eat this one sparingly, and only on rare occasions.) Add to the bean foundation a mixture of lettuce, onions, and tomatoes and a bit of salsa (which is hot and salty but oil-free). Remember to tell the server that you want no cheese, no sour cream, no olives, and no avocado (or guacamole) on your bean burrito.

Chinese foods: If possible, find a place that serves whole-grain brown rice. White rice is close enough, but it lacks fiber and nutrients, so the brown is preferred. Along with your rice (whether brown or white), ask for vegetables cooked in a "light" sauce that contains no oil or MSG. Beware of the hot mustard found on the table—it contains oil from the mustard seeds (and it can incinerate your tonsils). And watch for MSG in the soy sauce. Many Chinese restaurants now advertise in the telephone directory that they cook without MSG or oil on request.

Japanese foods: Ask the server about the cooked dishes the chef can make for you from vegetables, but without oil. One of these treats is rice topped with finely sliced vegetables that have been slightly cooked in a light ginger sauce. If the restaurant has a sushi bar, you're definitely in luck. You can always order sushi made of rice rolled in seaweed with a central core of raw cucumber and other vegetables (*kappamaki*). Sometimes the sushi contains pickled daikon (*oshinkomaki*). The rice in the roll is white, but for all but the most sensitive eater, this occasional mild insult to your system need not be harmful. The hot green horseradish called *wasabi* does add a little oil to your meal, but not much, because you'll use so little of it (it's very hot). A mixture of soy sauce (no MSG) and hot green *wasabi* is traditional for Japanese sushi and gives the dominant accent regardless of what vegetables are inside the roll of rice. You can order pickled salads too. Look in the *tsukemono* section of the menu for a whole variety of salads featuring assorted pickled vegetables. A cucumber and carrot salad is especially delectable.

Thai foods: Try green papaya and cabbage salad, or sweet-and-sour vegetables over brown rice. Be careful: Thai food can be very hot, especially if you use the pepper sauce placed on every table. Ask the chef to fix you "mild" or "cool" dishes if you don't want them to be too spicy.

Indian foods: Ask the chef to prepare your vegetarian meal without oil and dairy products. Some of our favorite dishes are made with sauces of garbanzo beans and eggplant. These sauces are served over rice (whole-grain is preferable, but white will do). Specify how spicy you want your dish. Among the Indian foods we commonly order are *samosa* (stuffed bread pocket), *urid dal* (bean curry), *moong dal* (lentil curry), *pilao* (a rice dish), *chana masala* (garbanzo beans), *alu gobi* (cauliflower), *upma* (wheat and vegetables), *khichuri* (lentils and rice), *tel baigan* (eggplant curry), and *bhindi bhaji* (okra and onions).

Vegetarian or health food: You should be able to find whole-grain (brown) rice and steamed vegetables at any such restaurant. Ask about dishes made without oil, eggs, or dairy products. Just because a restaurant advertises health food, don't assume all the foods will be "thinning." Most such restaurants use copious amounts of fattening oils, dairy products, and eggs in their dishes—not much is available for the maximum-weight-loss program.

Italian foods: On the original McDougall Program, Italian foods, such as spaghetti and dairy-free pizza, were permitted. Seek out an Italian restaurant that uses egg-free noodles and ask whether you can order an oil-free marinara sauce. Some restaurants may even have an oil-free vegetarian minestrone soup.

For pizza, find a place that uses whole-wheat flour and little or no oil in the crust, and an oil-free tomato sauce. Be specific in your order of toppings. You want generous amounts of oil-less tomato sauce, followed by onions, green pepper, mushrooms, and/or tomatoes. No cheese. No pepperoni. "We make, you bake" shops are often good choices.

The Best of Fast Foods

Admit it. You like the convenience and the prices at fast-food restaurants. Before becoming health-conscious you probably enjoyed more than a few selections from their billboard menus. Are you now banned forever from ordering in a drive-through lane? Only if you can't resist the temptation of all that salt and grease. If you're willing to stop asking "Where's the beef?" and you really want to "have it your way," you're ready to venture safely past the golden arches into the inner sanctums of ultraconvenience.

The fat-free items you will find first at many fast-food establishments are table sugar, pancake syrup, and jelly. If you look around a bit more, you'll find a few healthful items available at most of these establishments. Fast-food chains have heard the consumers' demands and now offer more vegetarian entrees and side dishes.

Your best choices are the places that serve plain baked potatoes and have a salad bar. Wendy's and Carl's Jr. have baked potatoes. Eat them plain or order onions, chives, and/or salsa for toppings. You should feel especially good about this because when that potato becomes French fries or hash browns, it contains triple the calories and increases the fat from 1 percent to 45 percent.

Wendy's, Pizza Hut, and Sizzler are famous for bountiful salad bars. Choose plenty of fresh vegetables. Avoid all the oil and mayonnaise-laden items, such as the coleslaw at 46 percent fat and 40 milligrams of cholesterol per quarter-cup serving. Top your salad with two tablespoons of wine vinegar, which adds only four calories (and no fat or cholesterol), or with lemon juice. This is a much wiser choice than two tablespoons of blue-cheese dressing, which contains 300 calories, 512 milligrams of sodium, and 58 milligrams of cholesterol. An even tastier choice might be to bring your own no-oil salad dressing from home.

If the place doesn't have a salad bar, you'll usually find a "garden salad" you can modify—leaving off the cheese and egg reduces the calories from 112 to less than 50 and the cholesterol from 116 milligrams to 0.

Potatoes and salads are about all you're going to get at a fast-food place if you stick to the McDougall Program for Maximum Weight Loss. However, if you were to slip to the principles of the original McDougall Program, you would be able to add a few items that use flour. Sandwich shops offer you some healthy choices. Subway Sandwiches has whole-wheat bread rolls that can be stuffed with onions, tomatoes, green peppers, and lettuce. Skip the oily dressing and the mayonnaise. A thin spread of mustard at four calories per teaspoon will add more flavor than any oil can. Another up-and-coming sandwich chain, Togo's, also takes pride in its vegetable sandwiches. A few sandwich places have started to use no-oil salad dressings. The more vegetables on the sandwich, the more you are using the McDougall weight-loss principles.

As for other fast-food choices, pizza would not be an obvious choice for healthy fast food unless you order it without the cheese (and without meat). By leaving off the cheese on a large Round Table vegetarian pizza, you eliminate 1,135 calories and nearly 300 milligram of cholesterol. The pizza sauce is oil-free —made of tomatoes and spices (amounting to 110 calories on that large pizza). You can ask for extra tomato sauce. There is a small amount of vegetable fat and salt in the dough (7.6 percent fat). The best toppings are tomatoes, onions, green peppers, mushrooms, and pineapple. Be careful of olives on your pizza; they add large amounts of fat (they are 96 percent fat) and salt (10 black olives add 631 milligram of sodium). Round Table, Domino's, and Pizza Hut have all made tasty, very-low-fat pizzas for us in the recent past.

Fast-food bean burritos sound pretty harmless. After all, the ones you make at home are nutritionally sound (about 2 to 5 percent fat and as little as 20 milligrams of sodium, depending on the kind of burrito shell you choose). Some places, like Taco Bell, claim to be interested in your health and boast of using only vegetable oil in their beans and burrito shells. Unfortunately, the nutritional information supplied by the company discloses that fat accounts for about 26 percent of the calories, with 888 milligram of sodium per burrito. Leaving off the tiny glob of cheese is a worthwhile gesture for a healthier dinner at Taco Bell, but there is still plenty of vegetable oil left to plump up your thighs. Most other fast-food Mexican stands don't even make the effort to appear health-conscious. They load copious amounts of lard into their beans. But some Mexican places do have oil-free beans (usually cooked whole beans), so ask. At Burger King, you can order a "Veggie Whopper." It is important to add, "Leave off the mayonnaise—just tomatoes, lettuce, onions (and maybe a few pickles, mustard, and ketchup), please." White-bread buns are 10 percent fat, with trace cholesterol and 250 milligrams of sodium. You can order an array of vegetables between white-bread buns at any burger joint.

Eating at Someone's Home

Eating at someone else's house requires a delicate balance between upholding your principles (and good sense) and protecting your host's feelings. You can begin by explaining that you are on a special diet. You can say that you are "following doctor's orders" and can eat only whole grains, vegetables, and fruits. You can also offer to bring a dish for everyone to try. If you think you may not be able to resist the temptation of another person's food, eat at home before you go out. It will be much easier to be strong when your stomach is already nicely full.

Airplane Food

Traveling by air is no excuse to drop your diet. Call the airline twenty-four hours before takeoff to order a special meal. Any travel agent can include your preferences in meals in your computerized reservation file so that they are automatically ordered every time you schedule a flight. Ask for "pure-vegetarian, no-oil" meals or a fruit plate. On a domestic flight, carry your own food from home.

Conclusion

Many people complain that the world is not arranged to help people to eat healthfully. It's true that the standard American diet is poisonous, and if you go along with the crowd, you'll eat your way into obesity, sickness, and premature death. But you have the power to change all that; you have the power to make the world meet your needs. All you have to do is ask with clarity and specificity. You'll be amazed by what restaurants will provide you, happily, when you know what you want.

CHAPTER 15

Shopping and Food Preparation for the McDougall Program for Maximum Weight Loss

Begin by planning. Go over the recipes and sample menus below to find one or two selections you'll like for breakfast, lunch, and dinner. Pick a starch-based recipe for breakfast. Choose either a starch-based soup recipe or a starch-based salad recipe for lunch. If you want, you can have both. Add a dish from the very-low-calorie salad section. For dinner, pick one recipe from the main menu dishes and one recipe from the very-low-calorie salad section. For your snacks, pick from the very-low-calorie salad recipes. You can increase the weight-reducing quality of the diet by emphasizing the very-low-calorie salads. Have them throughout the day—as often as you like. You must balance the weight-reducing properties of the very-low-calorie salads with the greater satisfaction you will receive with starch-based recipes.

Only the moderate and rapid approaches for portioning can be recommended for most people. (See Chapter 6 for details.) Estimate your intake from starch-based meals and very-low-calorie salads by eyeballing the volume of the foods on the plate. Precise measurement with a scale or cup is unnecessary. Recipes for the salads and main dishes have been divided into serving sizes of approximately ten ounces. This does not mean you are to have only one serving from each recipe. You may easily require three or four servings at a meal from one or more recipes before you are satisfied. Remember, you are not to go hungry.

PORTIONING FOR MAXIMUM WEIGHT LOSS

Moderate approach—two-thirds starch and one-third very-low-calorie dishes

Rapid approach—one-half starch and one-half very-low-calorie dishes

Hasty approach—one-third starch and two-thirds very-low-calorie dishes

---

Sample Menus for Twenty-one Days

These are only suggestions. Please rearrange the menus in any way that appeals to you, and repeat meals as often as you like.

DAY 1

Breakfast: Potato Hash
Morning Snack: Raw Vegetables with Fresh Salsa
Lunch: Barley Mushroom Soup
Afternoon Snack: Rice Cakes
Dinner: Shredded Salad, Texan Vegetable Casserole
Evening Snack: Raw Vegetables with Oil-Free Dressing as a Dip

DAY 2

Breakfast: Couscous and Orange Cereal
Morning Snack: Corn Salad
Lunch: Summer Potato Salad
Afternoon Snack: Rice Cakes with Leftover Salad
Dinner: Spinach Salad, Garbanzo Stew
Evening Snack: Raw Vegetables with Eggplant Dip

DAY 3

Breakfast: Frozen Hash Brown Potatoes
Morning Snack: Rice Cakes
Lunch: Vegetable Soup
Afternoon Snack: Raw Vegetables with Tangy Garbanzo Dip
Dinner: Chunky Vegetable Salad, Wild Spinach Rice
Evening Snack: Rice Cakes Spread with Mushroom Dip

DAY 4

Breakfast: Baked Millet Breakfast Squares
Morning Snack: Raw Vegetables with Fresh Salsa
Lunch: Mexican Potato Salad
Afternoon Snack: Rice Cakes with Leftover Soup
Dinner: Tomato Vegetable Salad, Curry Stuffed Peppers
Evening Snack: Raw Vegetables with Tangy Garbanzo Dip

DAY 5

Breakfast: Puffed Rice Cereal
Morning Snack: One-Minute Coleslaw
Lunch: Vegetable Sweet Potato Chowder
Afternoon Snack: Rice Cakes with Leftover Salad
Dinner: Spaghetti Squash and Broccoli Salad, Potato Ratatouille
Evening Snack: Raw Vegetables with Fresh Salsa

DAY 6

Breakfast: Sweet Potato Beginnings
Morning Snack: Rice Cakes with Leftover Soup or Salad
Lunch: Fast Minestrone
Afternoon Snack: Raw Vegetables with Tangy Garbanzo Dip
Dinner: Zucchini Corn Salad, Mushrooms with Wild Rice
Evening Snack: Rice Cakes

DAY 7

Breakfast: Breakfast Apple Rice
Morning Snack: Cucumber Cilantro Salad
Lunch: Baja Soup

Afternoon Snack: Rice Cakes with Leftover Soup
Dinner: Oriental Green Salad, Vegetable Chili
Evening Snack: Raw Vegetables with Tangy Garbanzo Dip

DAY 8
Breakfast:.Oatmeal
Morning Snack: Zucchini Corn Salad
Lunch: Lentil Vegetable Soup
Afternoon Snack: Rice Cakes
Dinner: Green Bean Salad, Tex-Mex Potatoes
Evening Snack: Mexican Potato Salad

DAY 9
Breakfast: Potato Hash
Morning Snack: One-Minute Coleslaw
Lunch: Quinoa Salad
Afternoon Snack: Raw Vegetables with Fresh Salsa
Dinner: Cucumber and Watercress Salad, Bean, Squash, and Cabbage Soup
Evening Snack: Rice Cakes with Leftover Salad

DAY 10
Breakfast: Baked Millet Breakfast Squares
Morning Snack: Rice Cakes with Leftover Salad
Lunch: Garden Vegetable Soup
Afternoon Snack: Raw Vegetables with Dip
Dinner: Fast Spicy Slaw, Potato Medley
Evening Snack: Rice Cakes with Leftover Salad

DAY 11
Breakfast: Frozen Hash Brown Potatoes
Morning Snack: Cucumber and Watercress Salad
Lunch: Low-Cal Stew
Afternoon Snack: Rice Cakes with Leftover Salad
Dinner: Tostada Salad, Souper Salad
Evening Snack: Raw Vegetables with Tangy Garbanzo Dip

DAY 12
Breakfast: Puffed Corn Cereal
Morning Snack: Rice Cakes with Leftover Salad
Lunch: Allium Soup
Afternoon Snack: Raw Vegetables with Dip
Dinner: Chopped Broccoli Salad, Vegetable Rice Casserole
Evening Snack: Rice Cakes with Leftover Soup

DAY 13
Breakfast: Breakfast Apple Rice
Morning Snack: Raw Vegetables with Mushroom Dip
Lunch: Sprouted Lentil Salad
Afternoon Snack: Rice Cakes with Leftover Soup or Salad
Dinner: Creamy Garlic Soup, Thai Vegetable Salad
Evening Snack: Raw Vegetables with Sweet Pea Guacamole

DAY 14
Breakfast: Oatmeal or Seven-Grain Hot Cereal
Morning Snack: Raw Vegetables with Dip
Lunch: Curried Rice and Broccoli Salad
Afternoon Snack: Mini Rice Cakes with Eggplant or Mushroom Dip
Dinner: Festive Condiment Soup, Favorite Garden Vegetable Salad
Evening Snack: Rice Cakes with Leftover Soup or Salad

DAY 15
Breakfast: Frozen Hash Brown Potatoes
Morning Snack: Fast Spicy Slaw
Lunch: Green Potato Soup
Afternoon Snack: Raw Vegetables with Dip
Dinner: Jícama Salad, Sweet-and-Sour Vegetables
Evening Snack: Rice Cakes with Leftover Soup or Salad

DAY 16
Breakfast: Couscous and Orange Cereal
Morning Snack: Raw Vegetables with Dip
Lunch: Mixed Sprout Salad

Afternoon Snack: Rice Cakes with Leftover Soup
Dinner: Zucchini Slaw, Tomato Vegetable Sauce with Potatoes
Evening Snack: Bean and Rice Salad

DAY 17
Breakfast: Breakfast Apple Rice
Morning Snack: Rice Cakes
Lunch: Vegetable Barley Soup
Afternoon Snack: Raw Vegetables with Tangy Garbanzo Dip
Dinner: Greens and Vegetables, Potato Rice Medley
Evening Snack: Leftover Salad or Soup

DAY 18
Breakfast: Potato Hash
Morning Snack: Raw Vegetables with Dip
Lunch: Wild Rice Salad
Afternoon Snack: Sweet-and-Sour Salad
Dinner: Coleslaw, Potato Casserole
Evening Snack: Rice Cakes with Leftover Soup or Salad

DAY 19
Breakfast: Puffed Rice Cereal
Morning Snack: Leftover Salad
Lunch: Italian Potato Salad
Afternoon Snack: Rice Cakes with Leftover Soup
Dinner: Cucumber Salad, Mattar Guchi
Evening Snack: Raw Vegetables with Dip

DAY 20
Breakfast: Frozen Hash Brown Potatoes
Morning Snack: Raw Vegetables with Dip
Lunch: Grain Salad
Afternoon Snack: Rice Cakes with Leftover Soup or Salad
Dinner: Spicy Tomato Coleslaw, Savory Baked Vegetables
Evening Snack: Rice Cakes with Dips

DAY 21

Breakfast: Sweet Potato Beginnings
Morning Snack: Rice Cakes with Leftover Soup or Salad
Lunch: Curried Eggplant
Afternoon Snack: Raw Vegetables with Dip
Dinner: Twice-Baked Potatoes with Broccoli Mushroom Sauce,
Creamy Spinach Soup
Evening Snack: Rice Cakes with Leftover Soup or Salad

Make a Shopping List

Make a shopping list of the ingredients you don't already have around the house. There are some basic items you will want on hand. This list will help you stock your cupboards.

Nonperishable items you will need are listed as staples. If you don't already have these on hand, purchase them on your first trip to the supermarket and health-food store.

The quantities are based on what's needed for two people. If you are feeding more than two, check the recipes and adjust the quantities you purchase appropriately. Brand names of acceptable packaged and canned goods are listed on pages 179–91. Don't buy unacceptable foods if you want the diet to work.

STAPLES

Soy milk or rice milk (no-fat)
Lemon juice (bottled)
Sherry (optional)
Soy sauce (low-sodium)
Vinegar (white, wine, balsamic, rice, and cider)

Seasonings and Condiments

No-salt seasonings
Barbecue sauces (low-sodium, oil-free)
Mustard

Salad dressings (low-sodium, oil-free): Russian, Italian, French, etc.
Salsa (low-sodium, oil-free)
Tabasco
Tomato catsup (low-sodium)
Worcestershire sauce (no-anchovies variety)

Herbs (Dried) and Spices

Allspice
Basil
Bay leaves
Black pepper
Cayenne
Celery seed
Coriander (ground)
Chili powder
Cinnamon
Cumin (ground)
Cumin seeds
Curry powder
Dill
Garlic powder
Ginger (ground)
Italian seasoning blend
Mace
Marjoram
Mustard (dry)
Nutmeg
Onion powder
Oregano
Paprika
Parsley flakes
Rosemary
Red pepper (crushed flakes)
Tarragon
Thyme
Turmeric
White pepper

Beverages

> Cereal beverages (Postum, Cafix, etc.)
> Soda water or seltzer (no-salt)
> Herbal teas (no-caffeine)

General Shopping List

These are things I usually have available in my cupboard and freezer. Depending on which recipes you choose to make, some foods may need to be added to this general list.

> Several bags of assorted rice cakes
> One bag or box puffed cereal of your choice
> One 24-ounce box quick-cooking oatmeal
> One 21-ounce bag Seven-Grain Cereal or Hot Apple Granola
> One 16-ounce bag dry pinto beans
> One 16-ounce bag dry red kidney beans
> One 5-pound bag brown rice
> One 16-ounce bag millet
> One 16-ounce bag barley
> One 16-ounce bag green split peas
> One 16-ounce bag Great Northern beans
> One 16-ounce bag dry garbanzo beans
> One 16-ounce bag dry lentils
> One 16-ounce bag frozen green peas
> One 16-ounce bag frozen corn kernels
> One 24-ounce box frozen hash brown potatoes
> One box bulgur (cracked wheat)
> One box couscous
> Four 16-ounce cans low-sodium tomato puree
> Four 16-ounce cans low-sodium chopped tomatoes
> Four 8-ounce cans low-sodium tomato sauce
> Two 16-ounce cans black beans
> Two 16-ounce cans garbanzo beans
> Two 16-ounce cans white cannellini beans
> Two 16-ounce cans kidney beans
> One 16-ounce can pinto beans
> One 4-ounce jar chopped pimiento
> One 4-ounce can chopped green chilies

Fresh Ingredients

This is a general list of the fresh ingredients I usually purchase at the supermarket. With these fresh items, you have the beginnings of some of the unusual salads, soups, and main dishes found in this book.

2 heads garlic, or 1 jar crushed or minced garlic
1 piece fresh ginger
5 pounds small red potatoes
One 5-pound bag white potatoes
One 3-pound bag carrots
7 yellow onions
1 red onion
1 red bell pepper
4 green bell peppers
2 bunches scallions (also called green onions)
1 pound fresh mushrooms
1 bunch romaine
1 head iceberg lettuce
1 bunch green-leaf lettuce
1 bunch celery
4 to 6 tomatoes
2 cucumbers
4 zucchini
2 leeks
1 eggplant
1 large bunch broccoli
1 bag washed spinach
1 head cauliflower
1 box alfalfa sprouts
1 bunch radishes
1 lemon
1 bunch fresh parsley or cilantro
1 head cabbage
1 head red cabbage
1 orange
1 jícama
2 turnips
1 pint cherry tomatoes
2 pounds sweet potatoes
2 bananas
1 apple

Shopping at a Supermarket and a Natural-Food Store

With the list you have made for the week's menu, start at your local supermarket. Pick a market oriented to fresh fruits and vegetables. Many upscale markets have health-food and specialty sections where some of the unusual ingredients can be found.

You may need to shop in a natural-food store about once a month, stocking up on the items you cannot find in the supermarket. (A natural-food store emphasizes foods, not vitamin and mineral supplements and protein powders.)

Label Reading

The key to effective shopping is careful label reading. Ingredients are listed in descending order based on the amount in the package. Manufacturers can deceive you with food labels as they are currently regulated. Simple sugars, like sugar, corn syrup, fructose, and fruit concentrate, can be listed individually in order to move sugar from the first ingredient down the list.

Manufacturers have also found ways of hiding fats in the ingredient lists by calling the fats monoglycerides or diglycerides. You might recognize triglyceride as fat, but are likely to overlook the mono- and di-forms as some other kind of additive, unrelated to fat. The chemical difference among these three is the number of chains of fatty acid attached to the backbone (glycerol) molecule: one (mono), two (di), or three (tri). Lecithin is also a fat you may not recognize as such. Most lecithin is made from soybeans and is no more effective at lowering cholesterol than any other similar vegetable oil. You want to avoid fat as much as possible. Look for oils listed as ingredients on the label and avoid these products. You will often find one gram of fat listed in the nutritional breakdown on the label of an apparently low-fat product. This one gram represents the fat in the naturally low-fat vegetable food.

The Food and Drug Administration is in the process of improving labels so that you will be better able to judge the contents of a package. When you're buying packaged foods read the ingredient labels carefully, and reread them periodically to catch changes in manufacturing practices.

FIGURING PERCENT OF CALORIES

A little simple math will help you evaluate how much fat, protein, and carbohydrate is in a food or packaged product.

Percent of fat is calculated by multiplying grams of fat by *9 calories per gram*, dividing the answer (the number of calories of fat) by the total calories, then multiplying by 100 percent. Your goal is less than 10 percent fat.

Percent protein is calculated by multiplying grams of protein by *4 calories per gram*, dividing the answer (the number of calories of protein) by the total calories, then multiplying by 100 percent). Your goal is 7 to 15 percent protein.

Percent of carbohydrate is calculated by multiplying grams of carbohydrate by *4 calories per gram*, dividing the answer (the number of calories of carbohydrate) by the total calories, then multiplying by 100 percent. Your goal is more than 75 percent carbohydrate.

The McDougall Program for Maximum Weight Loss calls for less than 5 percent fat, 7 to 15 percent protein, and 75 to 90 percent carbohydrate.

A Shopping List: McDougall-Okayed Packaged and Canned Products

One of the toughest challenges you face when adopting a new dietary program is knowing what to buy when you enter the supermarket. You've already figured out that you'll be buying lots of whole grains, such as brown rice, barley, whole wheat, and oats, and lots of fresh vegetables and fruits. These are the easy foods. The tough decisions come when considering which packaged and canned foods to purchase. To help you with those choices, I have developed the following list of safe and approved foods. Each week, you can go over this approved roster and make your own shopping list. You can be sure that these foods are all part of the McDougall Program for Maximum Weight Loss and can be eaten within the guidelines laid out in Chapter 6. I have left in some items that should be used sparingly for flavoring. These salad dressings, barbecue sauces, spaghetti sauces, and catsups are made with simple sugars and/or processed fruits and vegetables.

The McDougall Program for Maximum Weight Loss can become almost effortless if you choose. You can find enough packaged grains and canned and frozen starchy vegetables to make your entire meal plan. With bottled sauces and salad dressings, you will be able to make an interesting, flavorful, colorful recipe in no time.

Here's the list.

McDougall-Okayed Packaged and Canned Products

MANUFACTURER/DISTRIBUTOR   VARIETY

Cold Cereals

These cereals are made with whole grains, are low in salt, sugar, and additives, and contain no added fats or oils.

U.S. Mills (Erewhon)	Crispy Brown Rice
Perky Foods	Crispy Brown Rice
Barbara's Bakery	Brown Rice Crisps
Arrowhead Mills	Puffed Wheat Puffed Rice Puffed Millet Puffed Corn

Hot Cereals

These cereals are made with whole grains, are low in salt, sugar, and additives, and contain no added fats or oils.

Mercantile Food Co.	American Prairie Organic Hot Cereals
Quaker Oats Co.	Quaker Oats Quick Quaker Oats

MANUFACTURER/DISTRIBUTOR   VARIETY

Hot Cereals (continued)

U.S. Mills (Erewhon)   Instant Oat Meal

Stone-Buhr Milling   Hot Apple Granola
                                 7-Grain Cereal

Golden Temple Bakery   Oat Bran

Barbara's Bakery   14 Grains

Arrowhead Mills   7 Grain
                                 Instant Oatmeal

Frozen Potatoes

These frozen potatoes have no added fats, oils, or salt. Most have sugar (dextrose) and a preservative added. (Mr. Dell's are potatoes only.)

Ore-Ida Foods   Hash Browns
                                 Potatoes O'Brien

Bel-Air   Hash Browns

Mr. Dell Foods   Hash Browns

J. R. Simplot Co.   Okray's Hash Brown Potato
                                 Patties

Popcorn

This means unprocessed popcorn (with no added ingredients). You can pop any natural popcorn yourself in an air popper or in the microwave.

H. J. Heinz Co.   Weight Watchers Microwave
                                 Popcorn

Nature's Best   Nature's Cuisine (natural
                                 popcorn)

Energy Food Factory   Poprice

Lapidus Popcorn Co.   Lite-Corn

Specialty Grain Co.   Pop-Lite Microwave Popcorn

Country Grown Foods   Gourmet Popcorn

Rice Cakes

These cakes are made of rice with other whole grains and seasonings, and have no added fats or oils. Some have added salt.

Quaker Oats Co.	Rice Cakes (lightly salted)
	Corn Cakes
	Caramel Corn Cakes
H. J. Heinz Co.	Chico San (Millet, Buckwheat, and more)
Hollywood Health Foods	Mini Rice Cakes (Teriyaki, Apple Cinnamon)
Pacific Rice Products	Mini Crispys (Apple Spice, Raisin N' Spice, Italian Spice, Natural Sodium Free)
Westbrae Natural Foods	Teriyaki Rice Cakes
Lundberg Family Farms	Rice Cakes (Wild Rice, Wehani, Brown Rice, Mochi Sweet)
	Brown Rice Chewies, Brown Rice Crunchies, Organic Brown Rice Mini Rice Cakes

Soups

These soups have no meat, dairy, or added fats or oils. Many are high in salt.

Dry Packaged

Nile Spice Foods	Cous-Cous (Tomato Minestrone, Lentil Curry, Lentil, Black Bean, Split Pea)
	Chili' n Beans
Wil-Pak Foods	Taste Adventure Soups (Black Bean, Curry Lentil, Split Pea, Red Bean)
Fantastic Foods	Fantastic Soups (Leapin Lentils Over Couscous, Fantastic Jumpin Black Beans, Fantastic Splittin' Peas, Pinto Beans and Rice Mexicana)

MANUFACTURER/DISTRIBUTOR	VARIETY

Soups (continued)

The Spice Hunter	Kasba Curry with Rice Bran Mediterraean Minestrone
Canned	
Health Valley	Fat-Free Soup (5 Bean, Vegetable and Country Corn, and Vegetable plus others)
Real Fresh	Andersen's Soup (Split Pea)
Hain Pure Food Co.	Fat Free Soup (Vegetarian Split Pea, Vegetarian Veggie Broth)
Mercantile Food Co.	American Prairie Vegetable Bean Soup
Trader Joe's	Mostly Unsplit Pea Soup

Dry Packaged Grains and Pastas

These grains contain whole grains only, with no added fats or oils.

Quinoa Corp.	Quinoa
Continental Mills	Ala—cracked wheat bulgur
Lundberg Family Farms	Rizcous (grain mixture—don't follow cooking directions—omit butter and olive oil)
Fantastic Foods	Brown Basmati Rice Whole Wheat Couscous
Arrowhead Mills	Wholegrain Teff Quick Brown Rice (Spanish Style, Vegetable Herb, and Wild Rice & Herbs)

MANUFACTURER/DISTRIBUTOR   VARIETY

Dry Packaged Grains and Pastas (continued)

Pritikin Systems

Pritikin Mexican Dinner Mix
Pritikin Brown Rice Pilaf

Near East Food Products

Spanish Rice
Wheat Pilaf
Taboule
Lentil Pilaf Mix

Sahara Natural Foods

Casbah-Wheat Pilaf
Casbah-Spanish Pilaf
Casbah Whole Wheat Couscous

Nile Spice Foods

Whole Wheat Couscous, Couscous
Salad Mix, Rozdali

Wil-Pak Foods

Taste Adventure (Black Bean
Flakes and Pinto Bean Flakes)

J. A. Sharwood & Co.

Sharwood's India Pilau Rice

Texmati Rice

Basmati Brown Rice

Tipiak

Couscous

Jerusalem Natural Foods

Jerusalem Tab-ooleh

Berhanu International Ltd.

Authentic Olde World—Lentils
Divine

Bean and Vegetable Dishes (Frozen or Refrigerated)

United Foods

Pictsweet Express Microwaveable
Vegetables

Bird's Eye, General Foods

Country Style Rice (microwave)

Canned and Bottled Bean and/or Vegetable Products

These products contain no added fats and oils and are low in sodium
and preservatives. The cans are made of metals that leach into the
foods unless they are coated. Glass jars, of course, contain no metal.

Eden Foods

Great Northern Beans (glass jars)
Pinto Beans (glass jars)
Adzuki Beans (glass jars)

MANUFACTURER/DISTRIBUTOR   VARIETY

Canned and Bottled Bean and/or Vegetable Products (continued)

Whole Earth	Baked Beans
Health Valley Foods	Boston Baked Beans
Hain Pure Food Co.	Spicy Vegetarian Homestyle Chili
Bush Bros. & Co.	Bush's Deluxe Vegetarian Beans
Brazos Products	Brazos Cajun Bean Dip
S & W Fine Foods	Maple Syrup Beans Deli-Style Bean Salad Mixed Bean Salad (bottled) Dill Garden Salad Succotash Garden Style Pasta Salad
Little Bear Organic Foods	Bearitos—Chili, Black Bean Dip
American Home Food Products	Salad Bar (Marinated Medley, Three Bean Salad, Garbanzo Beans, Kidney Beans)
Del Monte Foods	Dennison's Chili Beans in Chili Gravy
Beatrice/Hunt-Wesson	Rosarita No Fat Refried Beans
Guiltless Gourmet Walnut Acres	Bean Dips Garbanzo Beans, Pinto Beans
Stop & Shop Supermarket Co.	Chick-peas (garbanzo beans)
H. J. Heinz Co.	Vegetarian Beans in Tomato Sauce
Trader Joe's	Spicy Black Bean Dip

Canned Tomato Products

These products contain no added salt. If they are too bland, add salt at the table if your health permits. Metals leach from cans.

| Health Valley Foods | Tomato Sauce (coated lead-free
can) |

MANUFACTURER/DISTRIBUTOR   VARIETY

Canned Tomato Products (continued)

Del Monte USA	Tomato Sauce (No Salt Added)
	Original Style Stewed Tomatoes With Onions, Celery, Green Peppers (No Salt Added)
	Tomato Paste
Beatrice/Hunt-Wesson	No Salt Added Tomato Paste
	No Salt Added Tomato Sauce
	No Salt Added Stewed Tomatoes
	No Salt Added Whole Tomatoes
Contadina Foods	Tomato Puree
	Tomato Paste
Pet	Progresso (Tomato Paste, Tomato Puree)
Eden Foods	Crushed Tomatoes (No Salt Added)
Trader Joe's	Tomato Sauce
S & W Fine Foods	No-Salt Added Ready-Cut Peeled Tomatoes
Ital Trade, USA	Pomi (Strained Tomatoes, Chopped Tomatoes)
Walnut Acres	Tomato Puree
	Tomatoes

Salad Dressings

These contain no dairy products (whey, buttermilk, etc.), no fats, and no oils. Many state clearly *No oil*. Should also say *Low-sodium*.

Pritikin Systems	No-oil Dressing (Ranch, Tomato, Italian, Russian, Creamy Italian, etc.)
WM Reily & Co.	Herb Magic (All no-oil—Vinaigrette, Italian, Gypsy, Zesty Tomato, Creamy Cucumber)

MANUFACTURER/DISTRIBUTOR	VARIETY

Salad Dressings (continued)

American Health Products	El Molino Herbal Secrets (All no-oil—Herbs & Spices, etc.)
Kraft	Oil-Free Italian (high-salt)
H. J. Heinz Co.	Weight Watchers Dressing (Tomato Vinaigrette, French)
Cook's Classics	Cook's Classic Oil-Free Dressings (Italian Gusto, Country French, Garlic Gusto, Dijon, Dill)
St. Mary Glacier	Oil-Free Salad Dressing—many flavors
Trader Joe's	No Oil Dill & Garlic Dressing, Italian
Sweet Adelaide Enterprises	Paula's No Oil Dressing
Nature's Harvest	Oil-Free Vinaigrette, Oil-Free Herbal Splendor
Nakano USA	Seasoned Rice Vinegar
Uncle Grant's Foods	Uncle Grant's Salute—Honey Mustard Tarragon Dressing
S & W Fine Foods	Vintage Lites Oil-Free Dressing
Tres Classique	Grand Garlic Tomato & Herb French Dressing
The Mayhaw Tree	Vidalia Onion Vinegar

Salsas

These contain vegetable ingredients only, with no oils. Some have preservatives. Many have added sugar and/or salt.

Hain Pure Food Co.	Salsa
Pet	Old El Paso Salsa
Tree of Life	Salsa
Nabisco Brands	Ortega Green Chile Salsa

MANUFACTURER/DISTRIBUTOR	VARIETY

Salsas (continued)

Pace Foods	Picante Sauce
La Victoria Foods	Chili Dip Salsa Jalapena, etc.
Ventre Packing Co.	Enrico's Salsa
Guiltless Gourmet	Guiltless Gourmet Picante Sauce
Pritikin Systems	Salsa
Trader Joe's	Salsa Authentica & Salsa Verde
Nature's Harvest	Salsa

Spaghetti Sauce

These contain no meat, dairy products, or added oils or fats. Use sparingly.

Pure & Simple	Johnson's Spaghetti Sauce
Trader Joe's	Trader Giotto's Italian Garden Fresh Vegetable Spaghetti Sauce
Westbrae Natural Foods	Ci' Bella Pasta Sauce (no salt, no oil)
H. J. Heinz Co.	Weight Watchers Spaghetti Sauce with Mushrooms
Campbell Soup Co.	Healthy Request Marinara Sauce
S & W Fine Foods	Pasta Sauce
Pritikin Systems	Pritikin Spaghetti Sauce (Original, Chunky Garden Style)
Beatrice/Hunt-Wesson	Healthy Choice Spaghetti Sauce
Nature's Harvest	Rocket Pesto
Tree of Life	Fat-Free Pasta Sauce
Sonoma Gourmet	Tomato Caper Herb Sauce

Barbecue Sauces, Catsups, and Relishes

These contain no added fats or oils, but most have added salt and sugar. Some have preservatives. Use sparingly.

Beatrice/Hunt-Wesson	Hunt's All Natural Thick & Rich Barbecue Sauce
Ridg's Finer Foods	Bull's Eye Original Barbecue Sauce
Robbie's	Robbie's Sauce (Barbecue—mild & hot, Sweet & Sour Hawaiian Style)
	Ketchup
Hain Pure Food Co.	Catsup
Kingsford Products	K. C. Masterpiece Original Sauce
Mrs. Renfro's	Mrs. Renfro's Barbecue Sauce, Tomato Relish, Corn Relish, etc.
New Morning	Corn Relish
Westbrae Natural Foods	Fruit Sweetened Catsup
	Unsweetened Un-Ketchup
Health Valley Foods	Catch-Up Tomato Table Sauce
Ventre Packing Co.	Enrico's Ketchup
Pure & Simple	Johnson's Ketchup
Beatrice/Hunt-Wesson	No Salt Added Tomato Ketchup
The Mayhaw Tree	Barbeque Sauce
Tim's Gourmet Foods	Tim's Barbecue Sauce

Soy Sauces

These soy sauces contain no MSG. They are all high in sodium, but some are salt-reduced.

Kikkoman Foods	Lite Soy Sauce
Westbrae Natural Foods	Mild Soy Sauce
San-J International	Tamari Wheat Free Soy Sauce

MANUFACTURER/DISTRIBUTOR   VARIETY

Soy Sauces (continued)

Live Food Products	Bragg Liquid Aminos
Edward & Sons Trading Co.	Ginger Tamari

Other Sauces

These contain no oils, fats, or MSG. Many have salt and preservatives. Some are very spicy. Use sparingly.

Nabisco Brands	A1 Steak Sauce
Lea & Perrins	Lea & Perrins Steak Sauce HP Steak Sauce
Oak Hill Farms	Vidalia Onion Steak Sauce Three Pepper Lemon Hot Sauce
Reese Finer Foods	Old English Tavern Sauce
San-J International	Teriyaki Sauce
St. Giles Foods Ltd.	Matured Worcestershire Sauce
McIlhenny Co.	Tabasco
Gourmet Foods	Cajun Sunshine
Durkee-French Foods	Red Hot Sauce
Baumer Foods	Crystal Hot Sauce
B. F. Trappey's Sons	Red Devil Louisiana Hot Sauce
J. Sosnick & Son	Kosher Horseradish
Reese Finer Foods	Prepared Horseradish
Aylas Organics	Szechwan, Cajun, Curry Sauce
Edwards & Sons	Stir Krazy Vegetarian Worcestershire Sauce

Salt-Free Seasoning Mixtures

These mixes are made with no added salt but contain a small amount of natural sodium. They are made of dehydrated vegetables and spices. Watch for added salt and oils in any seasoning mixes you buy.

Alberto-Culver Co.	Mrs. Dash (Low Pepper–No Garlic, Extra Spicy, Original Blend, etc.)
Modern Products	Vegit-All Purpose Seasoning Onion Magic Natural Seasoning
Parsley Patch	Parsley Patch (All Purpose, Mexican Blend, etc.)
Maine Coast Sea Vegetables	Sea Seasonings (Dulse with Garlic, Nori with Ginger, etc.)
Estee Corp.	Seasoning Sense (Mexican, Italian)
Hain Pure Food Co.	Chili Seasoning Mix
Bernard Jensen Products	Broth or Seasoning Special Vegetable Mix

Acceptable Milk Substitutes

These are dairy-free and low in natural vegetable fat. They should not be used as beverages but on cereals and in cooking.

Grainaissance	Amazake Rice Drink
Health Valley Foods	Fat-Free Soy Moo

Hot Drinks

These contain no caffeine or strong herbs.

Many manufacturers	Non-caffeinated teas
Modern Products	Sipp
Libby, McNeill & Libby	Pero
Worthington Foods	Kaffree Roma
Richter Bros.	Cafix
General Foods Corp.	Postum

For an updated package list send a self-addressed, stamped envelope to:

McDougalls Package List
P.O. Box 14039
Santa Rosa, CA 95402

Cooking Techniques for the Maximum-Weight-Loss Program

Cooking Without Oil

Leaving out the oil improves the taste appeal of a recipe, but you must devise other cooking methods and ways to replace the moisture and other qualities the oil once provided. Almost all the recipes you start with will have oil in one form or another as a prominent ingredient.

To sauté implies the use of butter or oil. But the McDougall interpretation leaves out the oil and instead uses liquids that have taste but are healthful. Plain water makes an excellent sautéing liquid. It prevents the food from sticking to the pan and still allows your vegetables to brown and cook.

For more flavor try sautéing in:

Soy sauce (tamari)
Red or white wine (alcoholic or nonalcoholic)
Sherry (alcoholic or nonalcoholic)
Rice vinegar or balsamic vinegar
Tomato juice
Lemon or lime juice
Salsa
Worcestershire sauce (no-anchovies variety)

Herbs and spices such as fresh ginger, dry mustard, and garlic can be added to the above suggestions for even more flavor.

Browning Vegetables

Browned onions take on an excellent flavor and can be used alone or mixed with other vegetables to make a dish with a distinctive taste. To brown and flavor your foods, place 1½ cups of chopped onion in a large nonstick frying pan with 1 cup of water. Cook over medium heat, stirring occasionally, until the liquid evaporates and the onion sticks to the bottom of the pan. Continue to stir for a minute, then add another ½ cup of water, loosening the brown bits from the bottom of the pan. Cook until the liquid evaporates again. Repeat this procedure once or twice until the onion is as browned as you like. You can also use this technique to brown carrots, green peppers, garlic, potatoes, shallots, zucchini, and many other vegetables, alone or in a variety of combinations.

Choosing Cookware

Acceptable materials for cookware include glass, stainless steel, iron, nonstick-coated pans and bakeware (such as Dupont's Silverstone or Teflon), silicone-coated bakeware (such as Baker's Secret), and porcelain. Using nonstick-coated pans is an important and easy way to eliminate oil from your cooking.

When buying cookware you need to pay most attention to the surface your food contacts, because there will always be some interaction that causes your food to pick up molecules from the surface. Aluminum cookware should be avoided because of the possible association between aluminum ingestion and Alzheimer's disease. (If you're stuck with an aluminum saucepan, put holes in the bottom and plant flowers in it.) For cake pans, loaf pans, and baking sheets you can use parchment paper between the metal and your food. Parchment paper also keeps food from sticking to the surface of the pans. You can find it in most grocery stores. Parchment can also be used under aluminum foil to keep the aluminum from coming in contact with the food. Place a layer of parchment paper over the food in the baking dish, then cover with foil, turning the edges over the pan to hold in the steam.

RECOMMENDED COOKWARE

One 2-quart saucepan (stainless steel)
One 3-quart saucepan (stainless steel)
One 4-quart saucepan (stainless steel)
One 6-quart stockpot (stainless steel)
One 8-quart steamer/pasta cooker (stainless steel)
One 12-quart stockpot (stainless steel)
One griddle (nonstick)
One large frying pan (nonstick)
One electric wok (nonstick)
One 9¼ × 5¼-inch loaf pan (silicone-coated)
One 9 × 13 × 2-inch oblong baking pan (silicone-coated)
One 8 × 8 × 2-inch square baking pan (silicone-coated)
One muffin tin (silicone-coated)
Two baking trays (silicone-coated)
One 2-quart covered casserole dish (glass)
One 3-quart covered casserole dish (glass)
One 6-quart square covered casserole dish (glass)
Two 9 × 13-inch oblong uncovered baking dishes (glass)
One 7½ × 11¾-inch oblong uncovered baking dish (glass)

If vegetables stick while cooking in a pan or baking tray, let them cool five to ten minutes and they will loosen easily. Cooling will also loosen muffins from the cups.

Microwave or Conventional Oven

Since the introduction of microwave cooking, people have been suspicious of "nuked" food. However, tests on the food show excellent nutrient content and no significant increase in harmful by-products from microwave heating, when compared with conventional oven cooking. We use a microwave mostly for boiling a cup of water, reheating leftovers, thawing vegetables, and cooking potatoes because it is fast and convenient. Sauces, stews, casseroles, and vegetables cook well in a microwave. Less liquid is needed and the cooking time is reduced compared to oven cooking. You must stir or rotate foods often, and foods should be covered when microwaved to hold in steam and to cook faster without drying.

The greatest safety concern for microwaves is leakage of the radiation from damaged units. Inexpensive microwave testers are available in most department stores. Buy one and check your unit periodically.

Seasoning Foods for the Maximum-Weight-Loss Program

Use the recipes in this book and those in previous McDougall books as guidelines only. You may prefer more or less spice. Mary and I have learned about individual tastes through years of counseling people. One person would tell Mary, "Your food is so bland, every time I make a recipe I have to double the spice." The next person would ask Mary why she uses so much spice. Mary has tried to flavor the foods to satisfy the average palate. (However, this moderate seasoning approach is subject to Mary's interpretation; for example, she happens to love curry and I do not. Fortunately, over the years my tastes have changed, and now I enjoy many of her Indian and Thai dishes.)

When deciding whether to use fresh herbs or dried ones in a recipe, consider how long the food is going to cook. If the cooking time is long, dried herbs are generally used. If the cooking time is short, use fresh herbs, if available. For equal flavor you will need more fresh herbs than dried ones because the dried ones are more concentrated. However, in time dried herbs lose their potency.

Particular combinations of spices are identified with various kinds of ethnic cooking. You can take advantage of these spices to vary recipes and create new ones.

Mexican	*Italian*	*Asian*
Salsa	Parsley	Soy sauce
Chili powder	Basil	Fresh ginger
Cumin	Oregano	Dry mustard
Cilantro	Garlic	Garlic

Greek	*Indian*
Lemon juice	Turmeric
Cinnamon	Curry powder
Cumin	Cilantro
Black pepper	Cumin

Place the Salt Shaker on the Table

Salt is the taste missed most when people switch to a healthful diet. If you think your food is bland, salt is what you are missing. Even if you never salted your food in the past, the amount in the prepared and packaged food you used to eat is substantially more than the 100 to 300 milligrams daily in an unsalted starch-based diet. The way to improve the taste is to add salt so that the salt-appreciating taste buds on the tip of your tongue will be delightfully stimulated.

The best way to keep your salt intake under control is to avoid, as much as possible, cooking with salt. Salt sprinkled on the surface of the food comes in contact with the tongue, providing the greatest pleasure for the smallest amount used. A few light sprinkles of salt will be enough for most people. Each half teaspoon of salt adds only 1,150 milligrams of sodium. This generous amount used daily will please most people's palates. Altogether this amounts to a total of 1,450 milligrams a day, 550 milligrams below the 2,000-milligram "low-sodium" diet served to patients in your community hospital's intensive-care unit. To bring the sodium intake up to the average of more than 5,000 milligrams used daily by most Americans, you would have to pour more than two teaspoons of salt on the surface of your starch-based meals daily. This amount of salt would render the food unpalatable for most people.

If your food still tastes a little bland, be patient—you will soon adjust to less salt and new flavors. Appreciation of the salty taste of foods is a learned behavior. Enjoying a lower salt intake is simply a matter of changing your habitual use and exposing your taste buds to lesser amounts. Adjustment begins in about four days.

Most of the recipes are deliciously seasoned and will not

need any salt added in cooking or at the table, especially after your palate has adjusted.

The recipes do not call specifically for low-sodium tomato products because most people can tolerate the amount of sodium used in canning. However, if you are salt-sensitive you will need to purchase the low-sodium varieties. For salt-free alternatives, use chopped fresh tomatoes in place of canned tomatoes, and in place of tomato sauce blend fresh tomatoes in a blender.

Soy Sauce

Soy sauce provides a flavorful alternative to plain table salt. Don't be fooled into thinking there is no sodium in soy sauce. The regular variety has 800 milligrams of sodium per tablespoon; the reduced-salt-varieties have 500 milligrams per tablespoon. When choosing a soy sauce, avoid monosodium glutamate. Many people have allergic reactions to this substance, and it represents another source of sodium. Soy sauce is also sold under the name tamari. There are variations in the taste of soy sauces depending on the manufacturer. You will likely develop a preference for one brand.

Notes on Sweeteners

Sweetness is the other pleasurable taste appreciated by the sensory buds on the tip of the tongue. You may wish to take advantage of this by adding a small amount of sweetener to the surface of your oatmeal. A teaspoon of sugar amounts to only sixteen calories.*

* A sugar is a sugar. There is little difference in nutritional impact among honey, maple syrup, molasses, brown sugar, and white sugar. They are all simple carbohydrates, best described as "empty calories." They contain no fiber, protein, or fat and contribute little or nothing to vitamin and mineral needs. Artificial sweeteners have their drawbacks too. They cause unpleasant reactions, such as headaches in some sensitive people. A few people claim even more severe reactions. The tastes of artificial sweeteners are not as pleasant as those of natural sugars. When you understand that sugar is a minor health hazard unless used in very large amounts, you realize there is little reason to resort to artificial sweeteners.

If you like (and if you tolerate them without adverse effects) you can use artificial sweeteners, but I see little advantage to them, since sugar used in reasonable amounts is not the cause of obesity or poor health. If you do use artificial sweeteners, apply them to the surface of your food for maximum taste.

Have Favorite Condiments on the Table

Having the right condiment or prepared sauce on the table can save the meal for family members not yet ecstatic about the new foods. Take advantage of the enjoyment provided by traditional sauces. (Make your own or select from the many sauces in the "McDougall-Okayed Packaged and Canned Products" list on pages 179 to 191.)

Success with the McDougall Maximum-Weight-Loss Program

Success comes from experience and experimenting. This may all be new to you and take some time for adjustment. However, after three or four days of sincere effort, most people adjust to the program. The benefit of eating to the full satisfaction of your appetite is one of the main reasons you will be able to adjust easily and permanently to this program.

CHAPTER 16

Recipes for the McDougall Program for Maximum Weight Loss

The following recipes were designed to help you lose the maximum amount of weight in the shortest time without going hungry or sacrificing your health. In fact, following this program will bring about dramatic improvements in your health. Which brings me to remind you again: If you are ill or on medication, you need to see your doctor before starting the program. Diet is powerful medicine, and your drugs will likely have to be reduced or discontinued. (See previous McDougall books for help, especially *McDougall's Medicine: A Challenging Second Opinion* and *The McDougall Program: 12 Days to Dynamic Health*.)

The recipes are divided into categories based on their use. Breakfast is centered around various starches. Lunch can be a soup or a grain salad, or both. For dinner, plan a starch-based main dish, along with a low-calorie salad. Salads are preferred for between-meal snacks because their use encourages maximum benefit from the program. However, the other starch-based selections are low enough in calories and fat that they will still work for most people as snacks.

The individual servings for the salads and main dishes are approximately ten ounces. The dressings and dips are provided in smaller portions. However, this does not mean that you are to limit yourself to one serving. You are encouraged to eat to the full satisfaction of your appetite. This means that at some meals you may eat three or four servings of a particular dish.

If you're not losing as quickly as you would like, you can do two things. First, increase your exercise. Second, increase your portions of low-calorie salads. However, you must keep satisfaction of your hunger drive in mind. The low-calorie salads are far less satisfying for most appetites than the starch-based dishes. Do not go hungry to hurry weight loss. As I have explained, this kind of suffering will not lead to permanent control of your health and appearance.

Once you have reached your goals you will want to explore the recipes designed for the original McDougall Program. You can find them in *The McDougall Program: 12 Days to Dynamic Health, The New McDougall Cookbook, The McDougall Plan,* and *The McDougall Health-Supporting Cookbooks,* Volumes I and II. (See Appendix for a list of recipes.) By this time you will be familiar enough with the principles of healthful eating that you will be designing your own recipes.

In Chapter 15, I presented a twenty-one-day menu plan. Some people like this kind of structure. However, most people will find the daily suggestions useful as just that—suggestions. You should design your own daily menus using the foods and spices you already enjoy and the time and desire you have to cook. If you are interested in saving time on food preparation, you will want to look over carefully the section on packaged and canned foods in Chapter 15. There you will find enough packaged grains and canned and frozen starchy vegetables to make up your whole daily diet. The bottled sauces and salad dressings will add all the flavor you could ever want to these starchy foundations. Most of you will develop a meal plan that combines the prepared products and the dishes you make from scratch.

Most people eat very simply and repeat their favorites over and over again. This kind of monotony makes life easier, and has some weight-loss and health advantages. Less variety in foods results in lower calorie intake and less chance of having an adverse (possibly allergic) reaction to food.

Don't forget to change the spices in the recipes to those you like, in the amounts you like. Also remember that most people in good health can add small amounts of salt (or soy sauce) to the surface of their foods. In no time at all you will have a collection of recipes that have become your all-time favorites, and you will be saying, "The more I eat, the healthier and thinner I get."

VERY-LOW-CALORIE GREEN AND YELLOW VEGETABLE DISHES

Favorite Garden Vegetable Salad

SERVINGS: 5
PREPARATION TIME: 30 MINUTES
COOKING TIME: 5 MINUTES (OPTIONAL)

8 cups torn leafy greens
(romaine, escarole, green
leaf, iceberg, etc.)
1 cup broccoli florets
1 cup cauliflower florets
1 cup diced zucchini
1 cup diced yellow
crookneck squash

1 cup diced red bell pepper
1 cup snow peas
1 cup cherry tomatoes,
halved
¾ cup oil-free salad
dressing

Wash, dry, and tear the lettuce into bite-sized pieces and place it in a large bowl.

Place all the vegetables except the tomatoes in a steamer basket and steam over boiling water 5 minutes. (This is an optional step. The vegetables can also be added to the salad raw for extra crunchiness and eye appeal.) Add the vegetables and tomatoes to the lettuce. Toss well to mix. Add the dressing and mix again. Serve at once.

Spinach Salad

SERVINGS: 2
PREPARATION TIME: 10 MINUTES

5 cups washed, torn fresh
spinach
1 small red onion, sliced
and separated into rings

1 seedless orange, peeled,
sliced, and quartered
⅓ cup oil-free dressing of
your choice

Combine the vegetables and the orange in a large bowl. Pour the dressing over and toss gently. Serve at once.

Variation: Add ½ cup sliced mushrooms to the other ingredients.

Hint: Use spinach from a bag of previously washed spinach to save time.

Cucumber Cilantro Salad

SERVINGS: 4
PREPARATION TIME: 15 MINUTES
CHILLING TIME: 1 HOUR

6 medium cucumbers
6 tablespoons lime juice
3 tablespoons chopped
fresh cilantro

1 tablespoon soy sauce
1 tablespoon chili powder
¾ teaspoon ground
coriander

Partly peel the cucumbers, but leave two or three strips of the skin on for color. Cut the cucumbers in half lengthwise, then cut in half lengthwise again. Chop into 1-inch pieces. (For variety, you can use sliced cucumber.) Place in a large bowl. Add the remaining ingredients and toss to mix. Chill for 1 hour before serving.

Bean Sprout Salad

SERVINGS: 6 TO 8
PREPARATION TIME: 30 MINUTES
CHILLING TIME: 8 HOURS

2 cups fresh green beans, steamed
1½ cups sliced cucumber
1 cup sliced celery
1 cup fresh mung bean sprouts
1 cup chopped green bell pepper

1 cup sliced mushroom
¼ cup chopped scallion
2 tablespoons chopped pimiento
1 cup oil-free dressing

Combine all the vegetables, tossing gently to mix. Pour the dressing over the top, toss again, cover, and refrigerate for 8 hours, stirring occasionally.

Greens and Vegetables

SERVINGS: 4
PREPARATION TIME: 25 MINUTES

1 cup torn romaine leaves
1 cup torn butter lettuce leaves
1 cup trimmed watercress
1 cup sliced fresh mushroom

1 cup sliced yellow squash
1 cup julienned zucchini
1 red bell pepper, sliced into thin strips
½ to ¾ cup oil-free dressing

Combine all the vegetables and greens. Mix well. Serve with your choice of oil-free dressing.

Chunky Vegetable Salad

SERVINGS: 4
PREPARATION TIME: 30 MINUTES
CHILLING TIME: 2 TO 4 HOURS

1 cup chopped fresh
tomato
1 cup sliced mushroom
1 cup chopped zucchini
1 cup chopped yellow
crookneck squash
½ cup chopped green bell
pepper
½ cup chopped red bell
pepper

½ cup chopped cucumber
½ cup shredded carrot
¼ cup chopped red onion
¼ cup finely chopped fresh
parsley
1 teaspoon finely chopped
fresh dill weed
½ cup oil-free Italian
dressing or another of
your choice

Combine all the ingredients in a large container with a cover. Shake well to mix. Refrigerate at least 2 hours to allow the flavors to blend; shake several times while chilling. This salad will keep several days in the refrigerator.

One-Minute Coleslaw

SERVINGS: 3
PREPARATION TIME: 1 MINUTE

One 16-ounce bag ready-to-
use coleslaw mix

One 8-ounce bottle oil-free
dressing

Open the bag of coleslaw and pour into a large bowl. Pour the oil-free dressing over the slaw and mix well. Serve at once, or cover and chill for use later.

Spaghetti Squash and Broccoli Salad

SERVINGS: 4
PREPARATION TIME: 30 MINUTES
COOKING TIME: 20 TO 25 MINUTES IN CONVENTIONAL OVEN,
20 MINUTES MICROWAVE
CHILLING TIME: 1 HOUR

1 medium spaghetti squash	1 tablespoon finely grated orange peel
2 cups chopped broccoli florets	½ cup seasoned rice vinegar
One 2½-ounce jar chopped pimiento	1 tablespoon soy sauce
Freshly ground pepper

To cook the spaghetti squash:

Conventional Oven: Pierce the squash several times with a fork. Bake in a 350°F oven for 45 minutes, turn over, and bake for another 20 to 25 minutes. Cool. Cut in half, remove the seeds, and pull out the cooked strands with a fork.

Microwave: Cut the squash in half and place cut side up in a baking dish with a small amount of water in the bottom. Cover tightly with plastic wrap. Cook on full power for 20 minutes, or until the skin is easily pierced with a fork. Let stand for 5 minutes. Uncover and cool. Remove the seeds and pull out the cooked strands with a fork.

Cooked squash can be covered and refrigerated up to 4 days.

For the salad, steam the broccoli until just tender. Remove from the heat, plunge into cold water, drain, and set aside.

Combine the spaghetti squash, broccoli, pimiento, and orange peel. Toss to mix. Combine the rice vinegar and soy sauce. Pour over the salad and mix again. This salad can be served at once or covered and chilled up to 1 hour. Season with freshly ground pepper before serving.

Zucchini Slaw

SERVINGS: 2
PREPARATION TIME: 15 MINUTES

2 small to medium
zucchini, julienned
2 small to medium yellow
straight-necked squash,
julienned
10 radishes, cut in half, then
thinly sliced
1 tablespoon chopped
fresh parsley

1 tablespoon chopped
fresh dill weed
⅓ cup Cook's Classics
Dijon oil-free dressing or
another of your choice
Freshly ground pepper to
taste

Combine all the ingredients and toss well to mix. This slaw can be served at once or refrigerated for later use. It still tastes great the next day.

Jícama Salad

SERVINGS: 6
PREPARATION TIME: 20 MINUTES
CHILLING TIME: 1 HOUR

1 small jícama, peeled and
diced
1 green bell pepper, diced
1 yellow bell pepper, diced

1 red onion, finely chopped
3 tomatoes, diced
1 cup oil-free Italian
dressing

Combine the vegetables in a large bowl. Pour the dressing over and toss to coat. Refrigerate for at least 1 hour to allow the flavors to blend.

Tomato Vegetable Salad

SERVINGS: 6
PREPARATION TIME: 30 MINUTES
CHILLING TIME: 1 TO 2 hours

6 tomatoes, chopped
2 cups fresh or frozen
   (thawed) corn kernels
2 zucchini, julienned
½ cucumber, finely chopped
½ cup water chestnuts,
   thinly sliced
4 shallots, finely chopped
1 tablespoon chopped
   fresh parsley

1 teaspoon chopped fresh
   basil
½ teaspoon minced fresh
   oregano
½ teaspoon minced fresh
   tarragon
½ cup oil-free dressing

Combine all the ingredients and toss well to mix. Chill before
serving.

Spinach Vegetable Salad

SERVINGS: 4
PREPARATION TIME: 30 MINUTES

6 cups loosely packed
   washed and dried fresh
   spinach leaves
½ pound mushrooms, sliced
2 carrots, thinly sliced

1 cucumber, thinly sliced
1 tomato, thinly sliced
1 cup alfalfa or clover
   sprouts
   Oil-free dressing to taste

Place all the ingredients in a large bowl and mix well. Serve
with your favorite oil-free dressing.

Thai Vegetable Salad

SERVINGS: 6 TO 8
PREPARATION TIME: 30 MINUTES

2 cloves garlic
2 to 4 small red chili peppers
or 1 or 2 teaspoons red
chili paste
6½ tablespoons fresh lime
juice
4 tablespoons soy sauce
7 cups finely shredded
cabbage

1 cup mung bean sprouts
1 cup shredded carrot
½ cup shredded daikon
½ cup chopped scallion
1 tomato, cut into thin
wedges, for garnish

Grind the garlic and chilies or chili paste in a small food processor.

Combine with the lime juice and soy sauce in a small jar. Cover and shake well to mix.

Combine the cabbage, bean sprouts, carrot, daikon, and scallion in a large bowl. Pour the dressing over and toss to mix well.

Garnish with the tomato wedges.

Cucumber and Watercress Salad

SERVINGS: 2
PREPARATION TIME: 10 MINUTES
CHILLING TIME: 30 MINUTES TO 1 HOUR

6 tablespoons white wine vinegar
1½ tablespoons water
4 tablespoons fresh lemon juice
3 teaspoons soy sauce

1½ teaspoons sugar
3 cucumbers, julienned
3 bunches scallions, chopped
3 bunches watercress, divided into sprigs

Mix the first five ingredients together. Set aside.

Add the cucumber and scallions to the dressing, tossing well to coat. Refrigerate until just before serving.

Wash the watercress well and spin or pat to dry. Place in a plastic bag and refrigerate until just before serving.

Before serving, combine the cucumber and scallions with the watercress. Toss to mix. Serve at once.

Shredded Salad

SERVINGS: 6 TO 8
PREPARATION TIME: 30 MINUTES

2 cups grated carrot
1 cup shredded red cabbage
1 cup grated zucchini
1 cup grated jícama
1 cup grated turnip
1 cup shredded romaine
1 cup torn spinach

½ cup sliced radishes
1 small red or mild white onion, sliced and separated into rings
½ cup oil-free dill dressing
Freshly ground pepper
1 cup cherry tomatoes, cut in half

Combine all the vegetables except the tomatoes in a large bowl. Pour the dressing over and toss to mix. Serve at once, garnished with pepper and the tomatoes.

Mixed Vegetable Salad

SERVINGS: 6
PREPARATION TIME: 30 MINUTES
COOKING TIME: 3 MINUTES
CHILLING TIME: 1 HOUR

1 cup frozen corn kernels
1 cup green beans,
  julienned
1 cup carrot, julienned
1 cup zucchini, julienned
1 cup yellow squash,
  julienned
1 cup red bell pepper,
  julienned

½ cup mild onion, cut in
  half and thinly sliced
1 cup oil-free salad
  dressing
Freshly ground pepper to
  taste

Bring a saucepan of water to a boil. Drop in the corn, beans, and carrot. Cook for 3 minutes. Drain and plunge into cold water. Drain again and place in a large bowl. Add the remaining ingredients and toss to mix well. Refrigerate for 1 hour before serving to allow the flavors to blend.

Fast Spicy Slaw

SERVINGS: 4
PREPARATION TIME: 10 MINUTES

2 to 4 small red chili
peppers
2 teaspoons crushed
garlic
¾ cup plus 1 tablespoon
fresh lime juice
½ cup plus 2
tablespoons soy sauce

2 teaspoons sugar
(optional)
Two 16-ounce bags ready-
to-use coleslaw mix

Grind the chili peppers in a small food processor. Mix with all the other ingredients except the coleslaw mix in a small jar. Shake well. Pour over the slaw mix and toss to mix well. Serve at once.

Coleslaw

SERVINGS: 4
PREPARATION TIME: 30 MINUTES
CHILLING TIME: 1 HOUR

DRESSING

2 tablespoons balsamic vinegar
6 tablespoons cider vinegar
2 tablespoons Dijon mustard
1 tablespoon soy sauce

2 teaspoons honey
½ teaspoon celery seeds
½ teaspoon caraway seeds
¼ teaspoon freshly ground pepper

SLAW

2 cups shredded green cabbage
2 cups shredded red cabbage
1 carrot, julienned
1 red bell pepper, julienned

1 yellow bell pepper, julienned
¼ cup finely chopped scallion
¼ cup minced fresh parsley
1 green bell pepper, julienned

Mix the dressing ingredients in a small jar and set aside.

Combine the vegetables in a large bowl. Pour the dressing over and toss to coat. Refrigerate for at least 1 hour to blend the flavors.

Sweet-and-Sour Salad

SERVINGS: 2
PREPARATION TIME: 15 MINUTES

DRESSING

3 tablespoons fresh lime
juice
1 tablespoon water
1 tablespoon finely
chopped fresh mint

1 teaspoon soy sauce
½ teaspoon honey
⅛ teaspoon ground cumin

SALAD

2 cups peeled and
julienned jícama

1 cup seedless grapes, cut
in half

Mix the dressing ingredients in a jar and set aside.

Combine the jícama and grapes. Pour the dressing over and toss to coat. Serve at once, or refrigerate until serving time.

Cucumber Salad

SERVINGS: 4
PREPARATION TIME: 5 MINUTES
CHILLING TIME: 1 HOUR

1 cucumber, cut in half
lengthwise and sliced
1 bunch scallions, sliced
One 15-ounce can sliced
bamboo shoots, drained
One 15-ounce can garbanzo
beans, drained and
rinsed

1 tablespoon brown sugar
1 tablespoon white wine
vinegar
Freshly ground pepper

Combine all the vegetables in a bowl. Combine the brown sugar and vinegar. Pour over the vegetables and toss to coat. Sprinkle with the pepper. Cover and chill for at least 1 hour.

Chopped Broccoli Salad

SERVINGS: 3
PREPARATION TIME: 20 MINUTES
CHILLING TIME: 1 TO 2 HOURS

DRESSING

1 small red chili pepper
½ teaspoon crushed garlic
3 tablespoons fresh lemon
juice

3 tablespoons soy sauce
½ teaspoon sugar (optional)

SALAD

1 pound broccoli, finely
chopped (about 4 cups)
½ cup chopped scallion

½ cup chopped roasted red
bell pepper

Grind the chili pepper in a small food processor. Mix with the other dressing ingredients and set aside.

Combine all the vegetables in a bowl. Pour the dressing over and mix well. Chill for at least 1 hour before serving.

Oriental Green Salad

SERVINGS: 2 TO 4
PREPARATION TIME: 15 MINUTES

1 cup torn leaf lettuce
1 cup torn Chinese
cabbage
1 cup mung bean sprouts
½ cup snow peas, trimmed

¼ cup thinly sliced celery
¼ cup broccoli florets
½ cup sliced canned
bamboo shoots
¼ cup thinly sliced carrot

3 tablespoons soy sauce	¼ teaspoon minced garlic
3 tablespoons rice vinegar	¼ teaspoon minced fresh
2 tablespoons water	ginger

Combine all the vegetables in a large bowl. Toss to mix. Set aside.

Combine the soy sauce, vinegar, water, garlic, and ginger in a blender. Blend briefly and pour over the vegetables. Toss to coat and serve at once.

Hint: This salad can also be served with your choice of oil-free dressing instead of the soy-sauce dressing given here.

Spicy Tomato Coleslaw

SERVINGS: 8
PREPARATION TIME: 25 MINUTES
CHILLING TIME: 2 HOURS

6 cups shredded cabbage	1 tomato, chopped
1 bunch scallions, cut into 2-inch pieces and then julienned	¾ cup spicy tomato juice
	¼ cup red wine vinegar
	1 tablespoon soy sauce
1 green bell pepper, julienned	½ teaspoon ground cumin
	¼ teaspoon freshly ground
1 cucumber, julienned	black pepper

Combine the vegetables in a large bowl. Set aside.

Pour the tomato juice and vinegar into a jar. Add the soy sauce, cumin, and pepper. Shake to mix well. Pour over the vegetables, tossing to mix. Cover and refrigerate for at least 2 hours to allow the flavors to blend.

Fresh Garden Salad

SERVINGS: 4
PREPARATION TIME: 30 MINUTES
COOKING TIME: 3 MINUTES
CHILLING TIME: 1 HOUR

1 cup julienned carrot
1 cup julienned green beans
1 cup fresh shelled green peas
1 cup julienned zucchini
1 cup julienned yellow crookneck squash

½ cup julienned jícama
½ cup julienned red bell pepper
½ cup finely chopped mild white onion
⅛ cup slivered fresh basil
1 cup oil-free dressing

Bring a large pot of water to a boil. Drop the carrot, beans, and peas into the water. Cook for 3 minutes. Drain, rinse in cold water, drain again, and place in a bowl. Add the remaining vegetables and mix. Add the dressing and toss to mix. Cover and refrigerate for at least 1 hour to allow the flavors to blend.

LOW-CALORIE DRESSINGS, DIPS, AND SAUCES

Raw Vegetables and Tangy Dips

SERVINGS: 4 TO 6
preparation time: 30 MINUTES

1 small bunch broccoli, cut into florets
1 small head cauliflower, cut into florets
1 cucumber, sliced
1 zucchini, cut into strips
1 carrot, cut into strips

1 or 2 stalks celery, cut into strips
Other vegetables of your choice, such as fresh green beans or asparagus

Prepare the vegetables and keep chilled for a quick snack. Serve with various dips as suggested below.

Fresh Salsa

SERVINGS: MAKES 2 CUPS

One 15-ounce can chopped tomatoes
½ small onion, coarsely chopped
¼ cup canned chopped green chilies

¼ cup tightly packed chopped fresh cilantro
1 clove garlic, minced (optional)
¼ teaspoon Tabasco

Place all the ingredients in a food processor or blender and process briefly until blended.

Tangy Garbanzo Dip

SERVINGS: MAKES 1½ CUPS

One 15-ounce can garbanzo
    beans, drained and
    rinsed
2 scallions, chopped
3 tablespoons water
2 tablespoons soy sauce

3 teaspoons grated fresh
    ginger
1 teaspoon rice vinegar
½ teaspoon honey
Dash or two Tabasco

Combine all the ingredients in a food processor or blender and process until smooth and creamy.

Sweet Pea Guacamole

SERVINGS: MAKES 2 CUPS
PREPARATION TIME: 15 MINUTES

2 pounds frozen peas,
    thawed
½ bunch cilantro, washed
    and trimmed
2 cloves garlic
¼ cup fresh lime or lemon
    juice

2 tablespoons rice vinegar
2 tablespoons soy sauce
1 teaspoon ground cumin
⅛ teaspoon crushed red
    pepper flakes (or to taste)

Combine all the ingredients in a food processor and process until fairly smooth.

Variation: For a chunky version of guacamole, stir in one chopped tomato and four chopped scallions.

"Cheese" Sauce

SERVINGS: MAKES 2 CUPS
PREPARATION TIME: 10 MINUTES
COOKING TIME: 10 MINUTES

¼ cup cooked, peeled
potato
2 cups water
One 4-ounce jar pimientos
½ teaspoon onion powder
¼ cup brewer's yeast
flakes (nutritional yeast)

3 tablespoons cornstarch
2 tablespoons fresh lemon
juice
Salt to taste, if desired

Blend the potato with ¼ to ⅓ cups of the water in a blender. Add the remaining ingredients and blend until smooth. Pour into a saucepan. Cook, stirring, until smooth and thick, 7 to 8 minutes.

Serve at once. The sauce will set when cool and can be reheated.

Tarragon Dressing

SERVINGS: MAKES 1¼ CUPS
PREPARATION TIME: 5 MINUTES

¼ cup apple juice
¼ cup fresh lemon juice
¼ cup balsamic vinegar
½ cup water

1 teaspoon minced garlic
1 tablespoon Dijon mustard
2 tablespoons dried
tarragon

Combine all the ingredients in a blender. Process until combined. Refrigerate at least 2 hours before serving.

Eggplant Dip

SERVINGS: MAKES 1¼ CUPS
PREPARATION TIME: 1 HOUR 10 MINUTES
CHILLING TIME: 1 TO 2 HOURS

Try this spicy dip with raw vegetables or mini rice cakes.

1 eggplant (1 to ½ pounds)
1 or 2 scallions, chopped
2 tablespoons minced fresh parsley
2 tablespoons minced fresh cilantro
1 teaspoon ground cumin
1 teaspoon ground coriander
½ teaspoon garlic powder
¼ teaspoon salt (optional)
Dash or two Tabasco

Cut the stem off the eggplant and prick it all over with a fork. Place directly on the oven rack and bake at 350°F for about 1 hour, until the eggplant is soft and has wrinkled skin. Remove from the oven and allow to cool. When it is cool enough to handle, peel and chop. Place in a blender with the scallions, parsley, and cilantro. Process until smooth. Place in a saucepan, add the remaining ingredients, and cook, stirring, until the mixture thickens slightly, about 10 minutes. Chill before serving.

Mushroom Dip

SERVINGS: MAKES 2 CUPS
PREPARATION TIME: 10 MINUTES
COOKING TIME: 12 MINUTES
CHILLING TIME: 1 TO 2 HOURS

Use as a dip for raw vegetables, or as a dip or spread for rice cakes.

1 pound mushrooms, chopped
1 cup washed, chopped leek
1 or 2 cloves garlic, minced
½ teaspoon dried oregano
½ teaspoon dried crumbled sage
½ teaspoon dried basil

¼ teaspoon poultry seasoning
1 teaspoon soy sauce
Freshly ground pepper to taste
¼ teaspoon prepared horseradish (optional)
Fresh lemon juice to taste (optional)

Place the mushrooms, leek, and garlic in a saucepan with a small amount of water. Sauté for 2 minutes, until the vegetables soften slightly. Add the remaining ingredients. Cook, uncovered, over low heat, stirring occasionally, 10 minutes. (Add a little more water if necessary to keep the mixture from sticking to the bottom of the pan.) Remove from the heat. Place in a blender or food processor and process until smooth. Chill before serving.

Citrus Dressing

SERVINGS: MAKES ⅓ CUP
PREPARATION TIME: 10 MINUTES

¼ cup fresh-squeezed
  orange juice
2 tablespoons fresh lime
  juice
1 tablespoon fresh
  cilantro, chopped and
  well packed

1 small clove garlic
½ teaspoon grated lime
  rind
1 to 4 drops Tabasco
⅛ teaspoon fennel seeds
  (optional)

Place all the ingredients in a blender and process until smooth.
Serve over fresh vegetable salads.

Tomato Dressing

SERVINGS: MAKES 1 CUP
PREPARATION TIME: 5 MINUTES
SETTING TIME: 1 TO 2 HOURS

¾ cup tomato, V-8, or spicy
  tomato juice
¼ cup red wine vinegar or
  balsamic vinegar
1 tablespoon chopped
  fresh parsley
1 tablespoon chopped
  chive or scallion

1 clove garlic, pressed
  (discard outer shell)
½ teaspoon salt (optional)
  Pinch dried oregano
  Pinch sugar
  Pinch ground cayenne
  Freshly ground pepper
¼ teaspoon guar gum

Combine all the ingredients in a jar and shake well to mix. Let
stand for 1 to 2 hours before serving to allow time for the guar
gum to thicken the dressing.

HIGH-CARBOHYDRATE, LOW-FAT BREAKFASTS, SOUPS, SALADS, AND MAIN DISHES

BREAKFASTS

Couscous and Orange Cereal

SERVINGS: 2
PREPARATION TIME: 10 MINUTES
COOKING TIME: 5 MINUTES

¾ cup water
½ cup couscous
2 oranges, peeled, sliced, seeded, and cut into quarters

1 tablespoon raisins (optional)
½ tablespoon honey
Dash or two ground cinnamon

Bring the water to a boil. Add the couscous, stir, cover, remove from the heat, and let stand for 5 minutes. Stir in the remaining ingredients. Serve warm.

Sweet Potato Beginnings

SERVINGS: 4
PREPARATION TIME: 10 MINUTES
(NEED COOKED SWEET POTATOES OR YAMS)

2 baked sweet potatoes or
  yams
2 bananas, sliced

1 apple, cored and chopped
½ teaspoon ground
  cinnamon

Peel and chop the sweet potatoes or yams. Combine with the bananas and apples. Mix well. Spoon into bowls and sprinkle each serving with cinnamon.

Breakfast Apple Rice

SERVINGS: 3
PREPARATION TIME: 10 MINUTES (NEED COOKED RICE)
COOKING TIME: 45 MINUTES OVEN, 10 MINUTES MICROWAVE

2 cups cooked brown rice
1 apple, cored and
  chopped
⅓ cup apple juice
¼ cup pure maple syrup

2 teaspoons fresh lemon
  juice
1 teaspoon vanilla extract
½ teaspoon ground
  cinnamon

Preheat the oven to 350°F.

Combine all the ingredients in a casserole dish with a cover. Bake in a conventional oven for 45 minutes or in a microwave oven for 10 minutes at full power, stirring once halfway through the cooking time. Serve hot.

Baked Millet Breakfast Squares

SERVINGS: 4
PREPARATION TIME: 15 MINUTES
COOKING TIME: 1 HOUR FOR MILLET, 45 MINUTES REFRIGERATION,
45 MINUTES TO BAKE

This recipe can be prepared ahead and reheated in the microwave if you like.

1 cup millet   ¼ teaspoon salt (optional)
4 cups water

Combine all the ingredients in a saucepan and bring to a boil. Cover and cook over low heat until the water is absorbed, about 1 hour.

Ladle into an oblong baking dish and flatten with a spatula. Refrigerate until set, at least 45 minutes or overnight. Preheat the oven to 350°F. Slice into ½-inch slices and bake on a nonstick baking sheet for about 45 minutes.

Serve warm topped with a small amount of unsweetened applesauce or fruit jam.

Cold Cereal Breakfast

SERVINGS: 1
PREPARATION TIME: 2 MINUTES

There are a few acceptable cold cereals on the market that are made from whole grains and have no added sugars or oils. They make for a fast, simple breakfast.

1 cup cold cereal   ¼ cup sliced bananas or
   Nonfat soy milk or rice   strawberries or whole
   milk   blueberries (optional)

Pour the cereal into a bowl. Add soy milk or rice milk and top with fruit, if desired.

Potato Hash

SERVINGS: 4
PREPARATION TIME: 20 MINUTES
COOKING TIME: 15 MINUTES

2 large potatoes, peeled and diced
1 medium onion, diced
1 green bell pepper, diced
1 red bell pepper, diced
1 cup frozen corn kernels, thawed

1 teaspoon poultry seasoning
¼ cup chopped fresh parsley or cilantro
Freshly ground pepper to taste

Cook the potatoes in water to cover until just tender, about 5 minutes. Drain and set aside.

Place the onion and green and red pepper in a saucepan with a small amount of water. Cook, stirring frequently, until just tender, about 4 minutes. Add corn and cook 1 additional minute. Remove from heat. Add the cooked potatoes, poultry seasoning, fresh parsley or cilantro, and pepper. Mix well.

Place the mixture in a large nonstick skillet. Cook, stirring frequently, over medium heat until the potatoes brown slightly, about 10 minutes. Serve with your favorite salsa or barbecue sauce.

Frozen Hash Brown Potatoes

SERVINGS: 1
PREPARATION TIME: 2 MINUTES
COOKING TIME: 20 TO 25 MINUTES

In the frozen food section of your supermarket you will find hash brown potatoes that contain shredded potatoes only or shredded potatoes with dextrose (sugar). They should not contain any oils. Different brands have different ingredients.

1 package frozen hash browns (use as many potato patties as you desire)

Place the frozen patties on a dry, nonstick griddle. Cook over medium to high heat for 15 minutes on the first side, then 10 minutes on the second side, until brown. Cover with catsup, oil-free barbecue sauce, or other acceptable favorites.

Hot Cereal

SERVINGS: 1
PREPARATION TIME: 2 MINUTES
COOKING TIME: 5 MINUTES

2 cups water
1 cup hot whole-grain cereal (seven-grain cereal, hot apple granola, or other)

Chopped fruit, such as bananas, apples, or pears

Bring the water to boil in a saucepan. Add the cereal. Stir, reduce the heat to low, and cook uncovered until done, about 5 minutes. Top with the fruit.

SOUPS

Vegetable Sweet Potato Chowder

SERVINGS: 6
PREPARATION TIME: 30 MINUTES
COOKING TIME: 50 MINUTES

3 cups frozen corn kernels
½ cup diced carrot
½ cup diced celery
½ cup diced onion
½ cup diced sweet potato
½ cup chopped tomato
¼ cup diced green bell pepper
¼ cup diced red bell pepper
1½ quarts vegetable stock or water

1 tablespoon soy sauce
½ teaspoon Tabasco
¼ teaspoon freshly ground pepper
½ teaspoon dried thyme
2 bay leaves
¼ cup cornstarch mixed in ¼ cup cold water
1 cup chopped fresh kale

Place the vegetables and stock or water in a large soup pot. Add the soy sauce and other seasonings. Bring to a boil, reduce the heat, cover, and simmer for about 45 minutes. Add the cornstarch mixture, stirring. Add the kale, stir, and cook another 5 minutes.

Garden Vegetable Soup

SERVINGS: 10
PREPARATION TIME: 20 MINUTES
COOKING TIME: 30 MINUTES

⅓ cup water
2 medium onions, chopped
2 medium red or yellow
  bell peppers, coarsely
  chopped
4 medium carrots, sliced
2 cups fresh corn kernels
  (cut from 2 ears of corn)
2 cloves garlic, minced
3 quarts vegetable broth
  (see Note)
2 zucchini, cut in half
  lengthwise, then sliced

2 yellow squash (straight-
  necked or crookneck),
  sliced
½ cup minced fresh parsley
  or cilantro
2 tablespoons minced fresh
  basil
2 tablespoons minced fresh
  oregano
Freshly ground pepper to
  taste

Place the water in a large soup pot. Add the onions, bell peppers, carrots, corn, and garlic. Cook, stirring, until the vegetables soften slightly, about 5 minutes. Add the vegetable broth. Bring to a boil, cover, reduce the heat, and simmer for 15 minutes. Add the remaining ingredients and cook for an additional 10 minutes.

Note: Make your own vegetable broth from recipes in other McDougall cookbooks (*The New McDougall Cookbook* has two recipes), or use canned vegetable broth available in natural-food stores and supermarkets, water seasoned with a small amount of soy sauce, or use half tomato juice and half water.

Fast Minestrone

SERVINGS: 10
PREPARATION TIME: 20 MINUTES
COOKING TIME: 1 HOUR

1 large onion, chopped
1 or 2 cloves garlic, minced
1 stalk celery, sliced
1 carrot, scrubbed and sliced
1 quart water
2 cups tomato juice
One 28-ounce can chopped tomatoes, with juice
1 potato, scrubbed and chopped
½ cup long-grain brown rice
1 tablespoon parsley flakes

1 teaspoon dried basil
1 teaspoon dried oregano
½ teaspoon ground marjoram
¼ teaspoon freshly ground pepper
1 zucchini, chopped
One 10-ounce package frozen chopped spinach
One 15½-ounce can cannellini beans

Place the onion, garlic, celery, and carrot in a large soup pot with about ½ cup of the water. Cook, stirring, over medium heat about 5 minutes. Add the remaining water, tomato juice, tomatoes, potato, rice, and seasonings. Bring to a boil, cover, reduce the heat, and simmer for 35 minutes. Add the remaining ingredients and cook for 20 minutes longer. Serve at once.

Vegetable Barley Soup

SERVINGS: 10
PREPARATION TIME: 20 MINUTES
COOKING TIME: 50 MINUTES

6 cups water or vegetable broth
½ cup uncooked barley
1 small onion, chopped
1 stalk celery, sliced
1 carrot, sliced
1 potato, peeled and cut into chunks
1 white turnip, peeled and cut into chunks

One 15-ounce can cannellini beans, drained and rinsed
1 bunch escarole or kale, coarsely chopped
1 or 2 tablespoons soy sauce
Freshly ground pepper to taste

Place the water or broth and the barley in a large soup pot. Bring to a boil. Add the onion, celery, carrot, potato, and turnip, stir well, reduce the heat, cover, and cook over low heat for 30 minutes. Add the beans and cook an additional 15 minutes. Add the greens, soy sauce, and pepper. Cook for another 2 or 3 minutes.

Variation: Add a washed, sliced leek along with the vegetables. Use two potatoes instead of the turnip, and add one chopped tomato along with the escarole and some fresh chopped parsley.

Vegetable Soup

SERVINGS: 10
PREPARATION TIME: 25 MINUTES
COOKING TIME: 40 MINUTES

1 onion, chopped
1 stalk celery, sliced
1 carrot, sliced
1 large potato, peeled and cut into chunks
2 large tomatoes, chopped
3 tablespoons chopped fresh basil
6 cups vegetable stock or water

2 small zucchini, cut in half lengthwise and sliced
2 cups cauliflower florets
1 cup frozen green peas, thawed
1 cup frozen corn kernels, thawed
2 tablespoons soy sauce
Freshly ground pepper to taste

Place a small amount of water in a large soup pot. Add the onion, celery, and carrot. Cook, stirring, over medium heat until the vegtables soften slightly, adding more water as necessary. Add the potato, tomatoes, basil, and stock or water. Bring to a boil, reduce the heat, cover, and cook about 15 minutes. Add the zucchini and cauliflower and cook for another 10 minutes. Add the peas, corn, soy sauce, and pepper. Cook for another 10 minutes, or until the vegetables are as tender as you like them.

Note: You can make your own vegetable stock from odds and ends of vegetables (see *The New McDougall Cookbook*) or use vegetable seasoning mix or vegetable stock sold in cans in natural-food stores and supermarkets.

Bean, Squash, and Cabbage Soup

SERVINGS: 9
PREPARATION TIME: 20 MINUTES
COOKING TIME: 30 MINUTES

1 cup chopped onion
½ cup chopped celery
2 cloves garlic, minced
½ cup water
1 cup chopped carrot
1 cup chopped winter
  squash
One 16-ounce can cannellini
  beans
3 cups vegetable stock
One 2-inch strip lemon peel
¼ teaspoon freshly
  ground pepper

⅛ teaspoon ground thyme
One 16-ounce can chopped
  tomatoes
4 cups shredded cabbage
1 teaspoon fresh lemon
  juice
½ cup chopped fresh
  basil
1 teaspoon grated lemon
  peel

Place the onion, celery, and garlic in a large soup pot with the water. Cook and stir until the onion softens slightly. Add the carrot, squash, beans, vegetable stock, strip of lemon peel, pepper, and thyme. Bring to a boil, reduce the heat, cover, and cook over low heat about 20 minutes. Add the tomatoes, cabbage, and lemon juice. Cook until the cabbage is tender, about 5 minutes. Stir in the basil and grated lemon peel.

Festive Condiment Soup

SERVINGS: 10
PREPARATION TIME: 40 MINUTES
COOKING TIME: 45 MINUTES

4 cups thinly sliced onion
8 cups water
3 tablespoons flour
One 16-ounce can tomato
  puree
1 clove garlic, crushed
1 tablespoon red wine
  vinegar
1 tablespoon
  Worcestershire sauce

1 tablespoon honey
½ teaspoon cumin seed,
  crushed
¼ teaspoon dried oregano
¼ teaspoon dried tarragon
¼ teaspoon freshly ground
  pepper
¼ teaspoon Tabasco
  Condiments: see next
  page

In a large pot, cook the onion in ½ cup of the water over medium-high heat, stirring often until a light brown glaze begins to form on the bottom of the pan. Add about ¼ cup more of the water and continue to cook the onion, stirring up all the browned bits.

Repeat this process two or three times until the onion is thoroughly cooked and a rich brown color. (This is important for flavor.)

Sprinkle the flour over the onions and stir. Add the tomato puree, the remaining 7 cups water, and all the remaining ingredients. Bring to a boil, reduce the heat, cover, and simmer over low heat for 30 minutes, stirring occasionally.

While the soup is cooking, assemble your choice of condiments from the list below. The more condiments you have available, the more festive the soup becomes. Have the condiments in individual bowls and let each person add whatever he or she likes.

CONDIMENTS

1 cup diced red or green
   bell pepper
1 cup diced cucumber
1 cup diced tomato
1 cup diced onion
½ pound mushrooms, sliced
   and sautéed in a little
   water

½ pound potatoes, boiled
   and chopped
½ pound carrots, sliced and
   steamed
1 cup cooked garbanzo
   beans
½ cup chopped fresh
   parsley

Green Potato Soup

SERVINGS: 6 TO 8
PREPARATION TIME: 20 MINUTES
COOKING TIME: 40 MINUTES

1 large onion, coarsely
   chopped
6 cups water
2 leeks, washed and sliced
   (white part only)
4 medium potatoes, peeled
   and coarsely chopped

¼ cup soy sauce
2 cups tightly packed
   washed and dried fresh
   spinach
Freshly ground pepper to
   taste

Place the onion in a large pot with ½ cup of the water. Cook, stirring, until the onion softens slightly. Add the remaining water, leeks, potatoes, and soy sauce. Bring to a boil. Reduce the heat, cover, and cook about 35 minutes. Add the spinach, stir well, and cook for another 2 minutes. Puree the soup in batches in a blender. Return to the pan and season with pepper.

Lentil Vegetable Soup

SERVINGS: 12
PREPARATION TIME: 20 MINUTES
COOKING TIME: 45 MINUTES

8 cups water
1½ cups dried lentils
1 onion, chopped
1 large carrot, chopped
1 celery stalk, chopped
2 potatoes, coarsely chopped, or 2 cups cooked brown rice
1 tablespoon chopped fresh parsley
1 teaspoon dried thyme
1 teaspoon freshly ground pepper

¼ teaspoon ground cloves
⅛ teaspoon liquid smoke
2 tablespoons water
2 tablespoons minced shallot
2 tablespoons minced garlic
1 teaspoon ground cumin
1 teaspoon ground coriander
Fresh parsley for garnish, if desired

Place the water in a large soup pot with the lentils, onion, carrot, celery, potatoes or rice, parsley, thyme, pepper, cloves, and liquid smoke. Bring to a boil, reduce the heat, cover, and simmer about 45 minutes.

Meanwhile, place the 2 tablespoons water, shallot, and garlic in a small pan. Cook, stirring, until tender, about 5 minutes. Mix in the cumin and coriander. Continue to cook, stirring, for another minute. Add to the soup and stir. Remove 3 cups of the soup to a blender. Puree until smooth and recombine with the rest of the soup.

Garnish with fresh parsley, if desired, before serving.

Creamy Garlic Soup

SERVINGS: 8
PREPARATION TIME: 30 MINUTES
COOKING TIME: 1 HOUR FOR GARLIC, 30 MINUTES FOR SOUP

2 whole heads garlic
2 medium onions, chopped
4 white potatoes, peeled and cut into chunks
5 cups water or vegetable broth

2 tablespoons soy sauce
Freshly ground pepper (optional)

Preheat the oven to 350°F.

Remove the loose papery skin from the garlic. Slice a thin strip off the top of the head and discard. Place the garlic in a dry baking dish and bake for 1 hour. Remove from the oven and set aside.

Place the onion in a large pot with a small amount of water. Cook, stirring, over medium heat until the onion softens slightly, about 3 minutes. Add the potatoes, water or broth, and soy sauce. Bring to a boil, cover, and simmer over low heat for 5 minutes.

Press the cooled garlic cloves out of the skins and discard all the skins. Add the garlic to the soup pot. Continue to cook for 25 minutes, until the potatoes are tender. Puree the soup in batches in a blender. Return to the pan and heat through. Season with pepper, if desired.

Allium Soup

SERVINGS: 12
PREPARATION TIME: 20 MINUTES
COOKING TIME: 1 HOUR

2 medium onions, cut in half and thinly sliced
2 or 3 leeks, washed and thinly sliced (white part only)
2 bunches scallions, chopped
2 or 3 cloves garlic, crushed
2 teaspoons minced fresh ginger
9 cups water
¼ cup soy sauce
Pinch ground cayenne
Freshly ground pepper to taste

Place the onions, leeks, scallions, garlic, and ginger in a large soup pot with 1 cup of the water. Cook, stirring, over medium heat for 5 minutes. Add the remaining ingredients, reduce the heat to low, cover, and cook for another 55 minutes to allow the flavors to blend.

Variation: For a heartier soup, add two potatoes, peeled and cut into chunks, when you add the remaining ingredients.

Souper Salad

SERVINGS: 8
PREPARATION TIME: 40 MINUTES
CHILLING TIME: 1 TO 2 HOURS

One 46-ounce can tomato juice
1 small red onion, finely chopped
1 clove garlic, minced
¼ cup water
½ cup fresh or frozen corn kernels
1 cucumber, seeded and finely chopped
1 red bell pepper, seeded and finely chopped
1 green bell pepper, seeded and finely chopped
1 zucchini, finely chopped
1 stalk celery, finely chopped

4 scallions, finely chopped
One 4-ounce can diced green chilies
1 cup finely chopped jícama
¼ cup chopped fresh cilantro or parsley
2 tablespoons red wine vinegar
2 tablespoons lime juice
1 tablespoon Tabasco
1 teaspoon prepared horseradish
Freshly ground pepper to taste

Pour the tomato juice into a large container. Place the onion and garlic and the ¼ cup water in a small saucepan. Cook, stirring, for 1 or 2 minutes, until the onion softens slightly. Add to the tomato juice. Add the remaining ingredients and stir well. Cover and refrigerate to allow the flavors to blend. This keeps for several days in the refrigerator. Stir before serving. Serve cold.

Hint: Add one 15-ounce can black beans, rinsed and drained —it adds more calories.

Creamy Spinach Soup

SERVINGS: 12
PREPARATION TIME: 20 MINUTES
COOKING TIME: 45 MINUTES

1 large onion, coarsely
  chopped
6 cups water
3 potatoes, peeled and
  chopped
3 zucchini, thickly sliced
1 tablespoon soy sauce

2 cups tightly packed
  washed and dried fresh
  spinach leaves
Several twists of freshly
  ground pepper
¼ package (3.5 ounces)
  enoki mushrooms
  (optional)

Place the onion in a large pot with ½ cup of the water. Cook and stir until the onion softens slightly, about 3 minutes. Add the remaining water and the potatoes, zucchini, and soy sauce. Bring to a boil, reduce the heat, cover, and simmer for 35 minutes. Add the spinach and pepper. Cook for another 2 minutes. Remove from the heat. Puree the soup in batches in a blender and return to the pan. Add the mushrooms, if desired. Heat gently for 5 minutes. Serve hot.

Baja Soup

SERVINGS: 12
PREPARATION TIME: 20 MINUTES
COOKING TIME: 50 MINUTES

4 cups water
1 cup salsa
1 medium onion, coarsely
  chopped

2 cloves garlic, crushed
1 green bell pepper,
  chopped
2 carrots, sliced

1 stalk celery, sliced
2 red potatoes, cut into
   chunks
1 cup fresh or frozen corn
   kernels

1 cup shredded cabbage
1 tomato, coarsely chopped
¼ cup chopped fresh
   cilantro (optional)

Place the first eight ingredients in a large soup pot. Bring to a boil, cover, and simmer for 30 minutes. Add the corn and cabbage. Cook for an additional 15 minutes. Add the tomato and heat through. Garnish with cilantro, if desired, just before serving.

Barley Mushroom Soup

SERVINGS: 4
PREPARATION TIME: 15 MINUTES
COOKING TIME: 1 HOUR

6½ cups water
½ cup barley
1 medium onion, chopped
1 tablespoon soy sauce
1 tablespoon parsley flakes
2 teaspoons dill weed
½ teaspoon ground cumin
¼ teaspoon garlic powder

⅛ teaspoon freshly ground
   pepper
⅛ teaspoon horseradish
   powder (wasabi)
½ pound mushrooms,
   sliced
2 cups shredded cabbage

Place the water, barley, onion, and seasonings in a large pot. Cover and cook over medium heat for 30 minutes. Add the mushrooms and cabbage and cook for another 30 minutes.

SALADS

Tostada Salad

SERVINGS: 12
PREPARATION TIME: 30 MINUTES
(NEED PREPARED GUACAMOLE AND SALSA)

1 cup fresh or frozen corn
kernels

1 cup diced zucchini

1 cup diced red or green
bell pepper

1 cup frozen peas

1 cup green beans, cut into
¼-inch pieces

1 recipe Fresh Salsa (see
page 217)

12 cups torn or shredded
lettuce (use a combination
of romaine, leafy green,
iceberg, etc.)

1 recipe Sweet Pea
Guacamole (see page 218)

Steam the corn, zucchini, pepper, peas, and beans for 5 minutes over boiling water. Remove from the heat, place in a bowl, stir in ⅓ cup of the salsa, and set aside.

To serve, place a mound of the lettuce on each plate, spoon the vegetable mixture over the lettuce, top with guacamole, and drizzle with the remaining salsa.

Note: Commercial oil-free bottled salsa may also be used. You can also find another good fat-free guacamole, called Broccomole, in *The New McDougall Cookbook*.

Green Bean Salad

SERVINGS: 4
PREPARATION TIME: 30 MINUTES
COOKING TIME: 30 MINUTES
MARINATING TIME: 1 HOUR
CHILLING TIME: 1 OR 2 HOURS

4 medium potatoes, cooked, peeled, and chopped (3½ cups)
4½ cups steamed fresh green beans
¼ cup oil-free Italian dressing
¼ cup balsamic or rice vinegar

2 or 3 cloves garlic
Freshly ground pepper to taste
Chopped fresh cilantro (optional)
1 small red onion, chopped

Measure ¾ cup of the potato and set aside. Combine the remaining potato with the green beans. Pour the oil-free dressing and vinegar over them, mix well, and allow to marinate for 1 hour.

Place the reserved ¾ cup of potato in a blender with the garlic. Process briefly and add small amounts of water until the mixture has a pastelike consistency. (The texture will vary depending on how soft the potato is.) Remove from the blender and place in a bowl. Stir in pepper to taste and the cilantro and onion. Stir this mixture into the beans and potato. Chill before serving.

Zucchini Corn Salad

SERVINGS: 6 TO 8
PREPARATION TIME: 15 MINUTES
CHILLING TIME: 1 HOUR

4 cups frozen corn kernels, thawed
4 cups julienned zucchini
4 scallions, sliced
2 tablespoons fresh lemon juice

1 tablespoon soy sauce
¼ teaspoon freshly ground pepper
¾ cup finely diced radishes
½ cup chopped fresh basil

Combine the first six ingredients in a bowl and toss well to mix. Add the radishes and basil. Mix gently. Cover and refrigerate for at least 1 hour before serving, but no longer than 3 hours to keep the radishes from discoloring.

Grain Salad

SERVINGS: 4
PREPARATION TIME: 10 MINUTES (NEED COOKED GRAINS)

3 cups cooked grains (see Note)
2 medium zucchini, halved and sliced
2 cups frozen corn kernels, thawed

¼ cup chopped scallion
¼ cup packed chopped fresh basil, dill, or cilantro
⅓ cup oil-free dressing

Combine the grains with the vegetables and mix well. Pour the dressing over the mixture and toss to combine. Serve at once or refrigerate for later use.

Note: The best grains for this salad are barley, rice, millet, and quinoa.

Bean and Rice Salad

SERVINGS: 8
PREPARATION TIME: 30 MINUTES (NEED COOKED RICE)
CHILLING TIME: 2 HOURS OR LONGER

4 cups cooked brown rice
One 15-ounce can black beans, rinsed and drained
One 15-ounce can garbanzo beans, rinsed and drained
½ cup chopped scallion
2 stalks celery, sliced
½ cup chopped green bell pepper
½ cup chopped red bell pepper
One 4-ounce can chopped green chilies
1 cup frozen corn kernels, thawed
1 cup frozen peas, thawed
¼ cup chopped fresh parsley or cilantro
1 cup of your favorite oil-free dressing or salsa

Combine all the ingredients in a large bowl and mix well. Cover and refrigerate for at least 2 hours to allow the flavors to blend.

Quinoa Salad

SERVINGS: 6
PREPARATION TIME: 15 MINUTES
COOKING TIME: 15 MINUTES
CHILLING TIME: 1 OR 2 HOURS

2 cups water
1 cup quinoa, rinsed well
2 cups chopped cucumber
1 cup chopped tomato
1 cup chopped green bell
    pepper
4 scallions, chopped
½ cup fresh lemon juice

2 tablespoons white wine
    vinegar
1 tablespoon soy sauce
4 tablespoons finely
    chopped fresh herbs (try
    basil, parsley, dill, and
    cilantro, varying each
    time for interest)

Bring the water to a boil in a saucepan and add the quinoa. Cover, reduce the heat, and simmer for 15 minutes. Remove from the heat. Let rest until all the liquid is absorbed. While the quinoa is cooking, prepare the other ingredients.

Combine the vegetables in a medium bowl. Add the quinoa and toss gently to mix.

Combine the lemon juice, vinegar, soy sauce, and your choice of fresh herbs. Pour over the salad and mix gently. Chill before serving.

Sabek's Tabouli

SERVINGS: 4
PREPARATION TIME: 1 HOUR
CHILLING TIME: 2 HOURS OR LONGER

2 cups boiling water
¾ cup bulgur
6 bunches fresh parsley,
   finely chopped
½ cup chopped fresh mint
1 bunch scallions, finely
   chopped

10 leaves romaine lettuce,
    finely chopped
¾ cup fresh lemon juice
2 tablespoons soy sauce

Pour the boiling water over the bulgur. Let stand for 1 hour. Put the bulgur in a mesh strainer and press out water. Put in a large bowl, add the remaining ingredients, and toss to mix well. Chill for at least 2 hours before serving.

Italian Potato Salad

SERVINGS: 4 TO 6
PREPARATION TIME: 20 MINUTES
COOKING TIME: 5 MINUTES
CHILLING TIME: 1 HOUR

5 large red potatoes,
   scrubbed and sliced ¼
   inch thick
½ pound mushrooms, sliced
1 small red onion, thinly
   sliced

½ cup chopped roasted red
   bell pepper
¾ cup oil-free Italian
   dressing
1 tablespoon chopped
   fresh basil

Drop the potatoes into boiling water and cook for 5 minutes. Drain. Combine with the remaining ingredients and toss well to mix. Refrigerate for 1 hour before serving.

Curried Rice and Broccoli Salad

SERVINGS: 6
PREPARATION TIME: 10 MINUTES (NEED COOKED RICE)
COOKING TIME: 5 MINUTES
CHILLING TIME: 1 HOUR

4 cups chopped broccoli
 florets
4 cups cooked brown rice
4 scallions, chopped
2 tablespoons fresh lemon
 juice
2 tablespoons water

1 tablespoon soy sauce
1 tablespoon balsamic
 vinegar
2 teaspoons curry powder
½ teaspoon ground cumin
¼ teaspoon freshly ground
 pepper

Steam the broccoli over boiling water until just tender, about 5 minutes. Rinse with cool water.

Combine the rice, broccoli, and scallions. Set aside.

Mix the remaining ingredients in a small jar. Shake to combine well. Pour over the rice and broccoli mixture. Stir to mix. Serve cold.

Wild Rice Salad

SERVINGS: 4
PREPARATION TIME: 15 MINUTES (NEED COOKED WILD RICE)

3 cups cooked wild rice
1 cup frozen corn kernels,
 thawed
2 chopped tomatoes
4 scallions, chopped
¼ bunch watercress,
 chopped (about 1 cup)

⅓ cup seasoned rice vinegar
½ tablespoon chopped
 fresh basil
Fresh greens

Combine all the ingredients except the greens and mix well. Serve on a bed of fresh greens.

Corn Salad

SERVINGS: 4
PREPARATION TIME: 15 MINUTES
COOKING TIME: 4 MINUTES

2 cups fresh or frozen corn
kernels (see Hint)
1 medium tomato, chopped
½ cup cooked kidney beans
(see Hint)
⅓ cup chopped green bell
pepper

⅓ cup chopped sweet onion
(Vidalia or Maui)
½ cup chopped mushrooms
¼ cup Cook's Classic Dijon
oil-free dressing
4 large lettuce leaves

Steam the corn until just tender, about 4 minutes. Combine with the remaining vegetables, except the lettuce leaves, and mix well. Add the dressing and toss again to mix. Spoon over the lettuce leaves and serve at once.

Hint: If you use fresh corn, steam or microwave it before cutting it off the cob. You can also use frozen corn. If you use canned kidney beans, rinse and drain them before adding to this recipe.

Summer Potato Salad

SERVINGS: 4
PREPARATION TIME: 10 MINUTES
COOKING TIME: 10 MINUTES

1 pound small red potatoes, quartered
2 cups zucchini, cut into chunks, or 2 cups halved Brussels sprouts, or 2 cups trimmed green beans

1 cup halved cherry tomatoes
2 scallions, chopped
½ cup oil-free dressing
1 teaspoon chopped fresh dill

Place the potatoes and zucchini, Brussels sprouts, or green beans in a saucepan with water to cover. Bring to a boil, reduce the heat, cover, and cook for 10 minutes, or until the vegetables are just tender. Drain. Place in a large bowl. Add the remaining ingredients, tossing gently to mix. Serve warm or cold.

Mexican Potato Salad

SERVINGS: 6 TO 8
PREPARATION TIME: 15 MINUTES (NEED PREPARED SALSA)
COOKING TIME: 30 MINUTES

2 pounds red potatoes, cut into chunks
1 cup frozen corn kernels, thawed
1 large tomato, chopped
1 bunch scallions, chopped
½ cup Fresh Salsa (see page 217)
2 tablespoons fresh lime juice
2 tablespoons chopped fresh cilantro or parsley
Freshly ground pepper

Place the potatoes in a large pot and cover with water. Bring to a boil, reduce the heat, cover, and cook 30 minutes, or until just tender. (Don't let them get too soft.) Remove from the heat, drain, and place in large bowl. Add the corn, tomato, and scallions. Combine the salsa and lime juice. Pour over the salad and mix well. Add the cilantro or parsley and a few twists of pepper. Mix gently and serve at once.

Variation: This salad can also be chilled before serving, and it is just as good the next day, so I always make lots of it.

Mixed Sprout Salad

SERVINGS: 4

PREPARATION TIME: 15 MINUTES (NEED SPROUTED BEANS)

CHILLING TIME: 1 HOUR

2 cups assorted sprouted
  beans (lentils, pea
  beans, adzuki beans,
  garbanzo beans, etc.)
4 scallions, sliced
6 mushrooms, sliced

6 to 8 cherry tomatoes, cut in
  half
1 stalk celery, sliced
2 tablespoons chopped
  watercress
⅓ cup oil-free dressing

Combine all the salad ingredients in a large bowl. Pour the dressing over and toss to mix well. Refrigerate for at least 1 hour before serving.

Sprouted Lentil Salad

SERVINGS: 4

PREPARATION TIME: 10 MINUTES (NEED SPROUTED LENTILS)

CHILLING TIME: 1 HOUR

4 cups sprouted red
  lentils
6 to 8 scallions, chopped
2 stalks celery, sliced
1 green bell pepper, cut
  into thin strips
One 4-ounce jar chopped
  pimientos

6 tablespoons chopped
  fresh parsley or cilantro
  cup oil-free salad
½ dressing

Combine all the ingredients in a large bowl and toss to mix well. Refrigerate before serving.

MAIN DISHES

Five-Grain Rice and Vegetables

SERVINGS: 8
PREPARATION TIME: 20 MINUTES
COOKING TIME: 1 HOUR FOR RICE, 30 MINUTES FOR CASSEROLE

3 cups water
1 cup Five-Grain Rice (see below)
1 medium onion, chopped
1 green or red bell pepper, chopped
2 medium zucchini, sliced
1 medium yellow summer squash, sliced

One 8-ounce can tomato sauce
1 clove garlic, crushed
1 tablespoon soy sauce
½ tablespoon chopped fresh basil
1 large tomato, sliced

Bring the water to a boil, stir in the Five-Grain Rice, reduce the heat, cover, and cook for 45 minutes. Remove from heat. Let stand undisturbed for 15 minutes. While the rice is cooking, prepare the other ingredients.

Place a small amount of water in a saucepan. Add the onion, bell pepper, zucchini, and squash. Cook, stirring until the vegetables soften slightly, about 5 minutes. Remove from the heat and set aside.

Combine the tomato sauce, garlic, soy sauce, and basil. Set aside.

Preheat the oven to 350°F.

Spread the Five-Grain Rice in the bottom of an oblong 10 × 6 × 8-inch baking dish, preferably nonstick. Spread the vegetable mixture over the grains and pour the tomato sauce mixture over the top. Finish with the tomato slices.

Cover with parchment paper, then top with foil, sealing the edges well. Bake for 30 minutes.

Five-Grain Rice

1 cup brown rice
¼ cup barley
¼ cup wheat berries
¼ cup millet

¼ cup whole rye, or ¼ cup
wild rice, or ⅛ cup of
each

Combine all the ingredients and store in a tightly covered jar. Use in recipes calling for rice or other whole grains.

Wild Spinach Rice

SERVINGS: 8
PREPARATION TIME: 30 MINUTES
COOKING TIME: 1 HOUR

3 cups water
1 cup long-grain brown
rice
½ cup wild rice
½ pound mushrooms,
sliced
1 bunch scallions,
chopped

1½ cups bean sprouts
1 pound fresh spinach,
washed and the stems
removed
2 tablespoons soy sauce

Place the water in a saucepan and bring to a boil. Add the long-grain rice and wild rice. Bring to a boil again, then reduce the heat, cover, and simmer for 45 minutes. Remove from the heat and let rest for 15 minutes.

Place the mushrooms and scallions in a large pan with a small amount of water. Cook and stir until tender, about 5 minutes. Stir in the bean sprouts and spinach, cover, and cook 3 or 4 minutes, until the spinach is wilted. Stir in the soy sauce. Add the cooked rice mixture and stir to combine. Serve with extra soy sauce for seasoning, if desired.

Vegetable Rice Casserole

SERVINGS: 10
PREPARATION TIME: 30 MINUTES (NEED COOKED RICE)
COOKING TIME: 30 MINUTES

1 pound broccoli, broken into florets
1 pound cauliflower, broken into florets
2 medium zucchini, sliced ½ inch thick
¼ cup sliced celery
¼ pound mushrooms, sliced
4 cups cooked brown rice
¼ cup shredded carrot
¼ cup chopped scallion
½ teaspoon soy sauce
1 cup mild salsa
20 cherry tomatoes, cut in half
1 cup "Cheese" Sauce (optional; recipe on page 219)

Preheat the oven to 350°F.

Steam the broccoli, cauliflower, zucchini, and celery over boiling water about 8 minutes. Add the mushrooms, and steam for 2 more minutes. Remove from the heat and set aside.

Mix the rice with the carrot, scallion, and soy sauce. Spread the mixture evenly in a 2-quart casserole or baking dish. Spoon the salsa over the rice and top with the steamed vegetables and tomatoes. Pour the "Cheese" Sauce over it all, if desired.

Bake, uncovered, for 15 to 20 minutes, until heated through.

Mushrooms with Wild Rice

SERVINGS: 4

PREPARATION TIME: 20 MINUTES

COOKING TIME: 1 HOUR FOR RICE, 30 MINUTES FOR VEGETABLES

1 cup wild rice
3 cups water
3 tablespoons soy sauce
¼ cup minced scallion
1 medium yellow onion, chopped
2 stalks celery, chopped
½ pound white mushrooms, sliced
8 fresh shiitake mushrooms, chopped

½ to ¾ cup chopped oyster mushrooms
½ teaspoon crushed dried sage
¼ teaspoon poultry seasoning
Freshly ground pepper to taste

Place the rice, water, 1 tablespoon of the soy sauce, and scallion in a saucepan with a tight-fitting lid. Bring to a boil, reduce the heat, cover, and cook over medium heat until the liquid has evaporated and the rice is tender, about 1 hour. Set aside.

Place the onion and celery in a large pan with about ¼ cup water. Cook, stirring, for several minutes, until the vegetables soften slightly. Add the mushrooms and cook, stirring occasionally, for another 10 minutes, Add the cooked rice and the remaining soy sauce and other seasonings. Cook over low heat for another 15 minutes.

Fried Rice

SERVINGS: 6
PREPARATION TIME: 15 MINUTES (NEED COOKED RICE)
COOKING TIME: 15 MINUTES

½ cup water
¼ teaspoon minced garlic
¼ teaspoon grated fresh
  ginger
6 cups mixed chopped
  vegetables (scallion,
  carrot, broccoli, bean
  sprouts, zucchini, etc.)

3 cups cooked brown rice
¼ cup soy sauce

Place the water, garlic, and ginger in a large pan or wok.
Heat to boiling. Add the vegetables and cook, stirring frequently, until the vegetables are tender-crisp, about 10 minutes. Add the rice and soy sauce. Mix well and heat through before serving.

Black-Eyed Peas

SERVINGS: 4
PREPARATION TIME: 10 MINUTES
SOAKING TIME: 12 HOURS
COOKING TIME: 30 MINUTES

1 pound black-eyed peas
1 onion, chopped
1 bay leaf

1 red bell pepper, chopped
2 tablespoons soy sauce
2 stalks celery, sliced

Soak the peas in enough water to cover overnight. Drain and put into a pot with the onion, bay leaf, red pepper, and soy sauce. Cover with water. Bring to a boil and cook for 20 minutes. Add the celery and cook for 4 or 5 minutes longer.

Potato Rice Medley

SERVINGS: 6
PREPARATION TIME: 15 MINUTES (NEED COOKED RICE AND POTATOES)
COOKING TIME: 15 MINUTES

1 medium onion, chopped
½ cup chopped red bell
  pepper
½ cup sliced mushrooms
½ cup fresh or frozen corn
  kernels
2 large white potatoes,
  cooked, peeled, and
  chopped

1 cup cooked brown rice
1 tablespoon soy sauce
1 tablespoon chopped fresh
  basil, or 1 teaspoon dried

Place a small amount of water in a large nonstick frying pan. Add the onion, pepper, and mushrooms. Cook, stirring frequently, for 5 minutes. Add the corn, potatoes, rice, and seasonings.

Cook, stirring frequently, until the potatoes and other vegetables are tender, about 10 minutes. (Add extra water if necessary to keep the vegetables from sticking to the bottom of the pan.)

Potato Casserole

SERVINGS: 6
PREPARATION TIME: 15 MINUTES
COOKING TIME: 1 HOUR

2 onions, sliced into
rings
1 or 2 cloves garlic, minced
½ cup water
One 16-ounce can chopped
tomatoes
One 8-ounce can tomato
sauce
½ teaspoon dried basil

½ teaspoon dried oregano
1 tablespoon parsley
flakes
¼ teaspoon freshly
ground pepper
1 tablespoon soy sauce
4 large white potatoes,
scrubbed and sliced

Preheat the oven to 350°F.

Place the onions and garlic in a medium saucepan with the water. Cook, stirring, over medium heat until the onion softens slightly and is easily separated into rings. Remove from the heat. Stir in the remaining ingredients except the potatoes.

Place a layer of the potato slices in a 9 × 13-inch nonstick baking pan. Cover with some of the tomato sauce. Repeat layers until all the potato is used, ending with a layer of tomato sauce. Place a sheet of parchment paper over the vegetables and cover with foil, sealing the edges tightly to keep in the heat.

Bake for 1 hour.

Dijon Mushroom Potatoes

SERVINGS: 4
PREPARATION TIME: 20 MINUTES
COOKING TIME: POTATOES: OVEN 1 HOUR, MICROWAVE 15 MINUTES
SAUCE: 20 MINUTES

4 medium baking potatoes, scrubbed
¾ cup water
1 onion, chopped
½ pound mushrooms, sliced
1 green bell pepper, chopped
1 small carrot, shredded
1 tablespoon soy sauce
1 tablespoon Dijon mustard
1 tablespoon cornstarch
Freshly ground pepper

Preheat the oven to 350°F. Prick potatoes in several places with a fork. Bake for 1 hour or until tender, or microwave on high power for 15 minutes, turning once. Let the potatoes rest while preparing the sauce.

In a large saucepan place ¼ cup of the water with the onion, mushrooms, green pepper, and carrot. Cook, stirring, until the vegetables are tender, adding a little more water if necessary.

Meanwhile, combine the remaining ingredients in a bowl. Stir into the vegetable mixture and cook, stirring, until thickened.

Serve the potatoes hot, passing the sauce separately.

Potato-Squash Boats

SERVINGS: 2
PREPARATION TIME: 15 MINUTES
COOKING TIME: OVEN 70 MINUTES, MICROWAVE 15 MINUTES

2 large baking potatoes
¾ cup chopped banana
    squash
⅛ teaspoon curry powder or
    ground cumin

½ teaspoon vegetable
    seasoning blend
Paprika

Preheat the oven to 425°F.

Scrub the potatoes and prick in several places with a fork. Bake until soft, about 1 hour or until tender, or microwave on high power for 15 minutes, turning once. Remove from the oven, cut in half lengthwise, and gently scrape the potato flesh from the skin, taking care not to tear the skin. (Leave ⅛ to ¼ inch of potato on the skin.)

Meanwhile, cook the squash in a small amount of water until soft, 10 to 15 minutes. Drain and set aside.

Preheat the broiler to low. Combine the potato pulp, cooked squash, curry or cumin, and vegetable seasoning blend. Mash with a potato masher until you have a creamy yellow puree. Spoon the puree into the potato shells. Sprinkle with paprika. Broil about 8 inches from the heat about 10 minutes, until lightly browned.

Potato Ratatouille

SERVINGS: 10
PREPARATION TIME: 20 MINUTES
COOKING TIME: 35 MINUTES

2 large yellow onions, chopped
2 cloves garlic, minced
¼ cup water
3 green bell peppers, chopped
4 zucchini, sliced
2 large potatoes, peeled and chopped
4 cups chopped tomatoes, fresh or canned
1 teaspoon chopped fresh basil
1 teaspoon chopped fresh oregano
2 tablespoons chopped fresh parsley
Freshly ground pepper to taste

Place the onions and garlic in a large pot with the water. Cook and stir about 3 minutes. Add the remaining ingredients except the pepper. Cover and cook over medium heat for 30 minutes, stirring occasionally. Season with the pepper before serving. This ratatouille can be served hot or cold.

Tex-Mex Potatoes

SERVINGS: 8
PREPARATION TIME: 20 MINUTES (NEED COOKED BEANS)
COOKING TIME: 40 MINUTES

6 firm red or white
potatoes
2 cups pinto beans,
mashed
1 cup Fresh Salsa (page
217)
One 4-ounce can diced green
chilies
1 small onion, chopped

1 clove garlic, crushed
3 tablespoons chopped
fresh cilantro
½ teaspoon chili powder
½ teaspoon ground cumin
1 tomato, chopped
¼ cup frozen corn kernels,
thawed
2 scallions, chopped

Preheat the oven to 375°F.

Scrub the potatoes and cut lengthwise into wedges. Place on a baking sheet and bake until lightly browned, about 40 minutes.

Meanwhile, combine the beans, salsa, chilies, onion, garlic, 2 tablespoons of the cilantro, chili powder, and cumin in a saucepan. Heat over very low heat about 15 minutes.

Combine the tomato, corn, scallions, and the remaining 1 tablespoon of cilantro. Set aside.

Place the potato wedges on a large serving platter. Spoon the bean mixture over the potatoes. Finish with the tomato and corn mixture.

Potato Medley

SERVINGS: 4
PREPARATION TIME: 10 MINUTES (NEED COOKED POTATOES)
COOKING TIME: 15 MINUTES

8 medium red potatoes, cooked

1 medium onion, coarsely chopped

½ pound mushrooms, sliced

10 stalks asparagus, cut into 1-inch pieces

1 cup tightly packed washed and dried fresh spinach

Chop the potatoes into large chunks. Combine with the onion in a large nonstick frying pan. Cook over medium heat for 5 minutes, stirring frequently. Add the mushrooms and asparagus. Cook, stirring frequently, for another 10 minutes. Add the spinach. Cook, stirring, just until the spinach wilts, another minute or so. Serve with a favorite sauce.

Easy Roasted Potatoes

SERVINGS: 4
PREPARATION TIME: 5 MINUTES
COOKING TIME: 1 HOUR

2 pounds red potatoes, cut into chunks

1 package Hain Onion Soup Mix

¼ cup water

Preheat the oven to 400°F.

Place all the ingredients in a large bowl with a tight-fitting lid. Shake well until the potatoes are coated with the soup mix. Transfer to a casserole dish with a cover. Bake for 30 minutes, stirring occasionally. Uncover and bake for an additional 30 minutes.

Twice-Baked Potatoes

SERVINGS: 4
PREPARATION TIME: 5 MINUTES
COOKING TIME: OVEN 1½ HOURS, MICROWAVE 15 MINUTES

2 large baking potatoes
1 scallion, chopped
2 tablespoons water
1 tablespoon fresh chopped
  parsley

Paprika
Freshly ground pepper

Preheat the oven to 425°F.

Scrub the potatoes and prick in several places with a fork. Bake until tender, 1 to 1¼ hours or in microwave on high power for 15 minutes, turning once. Reduce the oven to 400°F.

Cut a thin slice off each potato lengthwise. Carefully scoop out the insides of the potatoes and place in a bowl. Add the scallion, water, and parsley and mash until smooth.

Spoon the mixture back into the potato shells. Sprinkle paprika and pepper over the top. Place on baking sheet and bake for 15 minutes.

Vegetable Chili

SERVINGS: 8
PREPARATION TIME: 20 MINUTES
COOKING TIME: 40 MINUTES

½ cup water
½ cup chopped onion
½ cup chopped green bell pepper
½ cup zucchini, cut into chunks
½ cup yellow straight-necked squash, cut into chunks
1 cup frozen corn kernels
One 28-ounce can stewed tomatoes
1 cup cooked black beans
1 cup cooked pinto beans
1 cup cooked white beans
1 cup cooked garbanzo beans
¼ cup chopped green chilies
1 tablespoon chili powder
½ tablespoon soy sauce
Dash ground cayenne

Place the water, onion, and green pepper in a large soup pot. Cook and stir until the onion is tender, about 5 minutes. Add the remaining ingredients, stir to mix well, and bring to a boil.

Reduce the heat and cook uncovered over medium-low heat for 30 minutes. Serve in soup bowls by itself or over whole grains.

Italian Garbanzo Stew

SERVINGS: 8
PREPARATION TIME: 10 MINUTES
COOKING TIME: 32 MINUTES

1 large onion, chopped
1 large green bell pepper, chopped
1 or 2 cloves garlic, minced
One 28-ounce can chopped tomatoes
One 15-ounce can tomato sauce
Two 15-ounce cans garbanzo beans, drained

1 cup fresh or frozen corn kernels
1 teaspoon dried oregano
1 teaspoon dried basil
1 tablespoon soy sauce
Freshly ground pepper
2 cups packed washed and dried spinach leaves

Put the onion, green pepper, and garlic in a large pot with a small amount of water. Cook, stirring, until the vegetables are soft, about 10 minutes. Add the remaining ingredients except for the spinach. Mix well, cover, reduce the heat, and cook for 20 minutes. Stir in the spinach and cook until wilted, 1 or 2 minutes. Serve over rice or other whole grains.

Squashy Black Beans

SERVINGS: 4
PREPARATION TIME: 20 MINUTES
COOKING TIME: 15 to 20 MINUTES

2 cups winter squash, peeled and cut into chunks

2 medium onions, coarsely chopped

1 carrot, thinly sliced

1 stalk celery, thinly sliced

2 or 3 cloves garlic, minced

2 cups water

Two 15-ounce cans black beans, drained and rinsed

2 tablespoons chopped fresh cilantro

2 tablespoons soy sauce

2 teaspoons ground cumin

1 teaspoon grated fresh ginger

¼ teaspoon freshly ground pepper

Place the squash in a pan and cover with water. Bring to a boil, reduce the heat, cover, and cook for 8 to 10 minutes, until tender but not mushy. Drain and set aside. Meanwhile, place the onion, carrot, and celery in a large pot with ½ cup of the water. Cook over medium heat about 5 minutes, stirring occasionally, until the water evaporates. Add another ¼ cup of water and continue to cook, stirring, until that water evaporates. Repeat with another ¼ cup of water. After that water has evaporated, add the remaining water and other ingredients, along with the reserved squash. Mix well. Cook over low heat until the flavors are blended, about 5 minutes.

Serve over rice, whole grains, or potatoes.

Garbanzo Curry

SERVINGS: 6
PREPARATION TIME: 15 MINUTES
COOKING TIME: 40 MINUTES

1 medium onion, chopped
1 green bell pepper, chopped
⅓ cup water
1 teaspoon curry powder
½ teaspoon ground cumin
¼ teaspoon ground turmeric
¼ teaspoon freshly ground pepper
2 cups chopped red potato

2½ cups water
One 15-ounce can garbanzo beans, drained and rinsed
1 cup frozen green peas, thawed
1 tablespoon cornstarch mixed with 2 tablespoons cold water (optional)

Place the onion and green pepper in a large pot with the ⅓ cup water. Cook and stir until the onion softens slightly. Add the seasonings and stir to mix. Add the potato and the 2½ cups water. Cover and cook over low heat until the potato is tender, about 25 minutes. Add the beans and peas. Cook for an additional 10 minutes.

If desired, stir in the cornstarch mixture and cook, stirring until thickened. Serve as is or over whole grains.

Variation: Add 1 cup chopped green apple during the final 10 minutes of cooking.

Curry-Stuffed Peppers

SERVINGS: 6
PREPARATION TIME: 45 MINUTES
COOKING TIME: 1 HOUR

6 large bell peppers, red or green
2 pounds white potatoes, peeled and cut into chunks
⅓ cup finely chopped onion
1 cup chopped broccoli florets
¼ cup finely chopped carrot
¾ teaspoon curry powder
½ teaspoon ground cumin
½ teaspoon ground turmeric
½ teaspoon grated fresh ginger
1 tablespoon fresh lemon juice
1 tablespoon soy sauce
Freshly ground pepper

Cut the tops off the peppers and clean out the insides. Steam over boiling water for 10 minutes. Set aside.

Meanwhile, cook the potatoes in water to cover until tender, about 30 minutes. Drain, reserving the cooking water. Mash the potatoes, using a small amount of the cooking water to moisten. Set aside.

Preheat the oven to 350°F.

Sauté the onion in a small amount of the reserved potato water until translucent, about 3 minutes. Add the broccoli, carrot, curry powder, cumin, turmeric, and ginger. Cook, stirring for 3 more minutes, adding a little more potato water if necessary. Stir the vegetable mixture into the mashed potatoes. Add the lemon juice, soy sauce, and a few twists of pepper.

Stuff the peppers with the potato mixture. Place the peppers in a nonstick baking dish. Bake for 20 minutes. Serve with Curry Tomato Sauce (see the next page).

Curry Tomato Sauce

SERVINGS: MAKES 4 CUPS
PREPARATION TIME: 10 MINUTES
COOKING TIME: 10 MINUTES

1 bunch scallions, finely
  chopped
1 clove garlic, crushed
1 tablespoon grated fresh
  ginger

One 28-ounce can crushed
  tomatoes
¼ teaspoon curry powder
½ teaspoon ground
  turmeric

Place a small amount of water in a saucepan. Add the scallions, garlic, and ginger. Cook and stir over medium heat for a few minutes. Add the remaining ingredients. Mix well. Cook for another 6 or 7 minutes to allow the flavors to blend. Serve hot.

Tomato Vegetable Sauce

SERVINGS: MAKES 10 CUPS
PREPARATION TIME: 20 MINUTES
COOKING TIME: 1 HOUR

1 medium onion,
chopped
1 pound mushrooms,
sliced
1 clove garlic, minced
2 zucchini, sliced
1 red bell pepper,
chopped
One 28-ounce can crushed
tomatoes
One 15-ounce can chopped
or stewed tomatoes

One 15-ounce can tomato
sauce
¼ cup chopped fresh
parsley
Seasonings (see
Variations)
1 cup packed washed,
dried, and chopped
spinach

Place the onion, mushrooms, and garlic in a large pot with a small amount of water. Cook and stir over medium heat for 3 or 4 minutes. Add the zucchini, bell pepper, tomatoes, tomato sauce, and seasonings. Cook, uncovered, over medium-low heat for 1 hour. Stir in the chopped spinach. Cook just until the spinach wilts, about 2 to 3 minutes. Serve over potatoes or grains.

Variations: Italian: Add 1 teaspoon dried basil and 1 teaspoon dried oregano. Use Italian stewed tomatoes.

Cajun: Add 1 teaspoon dried basil and ½ teaspoon Tabasco. Use Cajun stewed tomatoes.

Mexican: Add 1 teaspoon dried basil and 1 teaspoon chili powder. Use Mexican stewed tomatoes.

Texan Vegetable Casserole

SERVINGS: 11
PREPARATION TIME: 40 MINUTES
COOKING TIME: 1 HOUR AND 35 MINUTES

1 medium eggplant, coarsely chopped
1 medium onion, coarsely chopped
2 stalks celery, thickly sliced
2 leeks, washed and thinly sliced (white part only)
2 cloves garlic, minced
4 red potatoes, coarsely chopped
1 green bell pepper, coarsely chopped
1 red bell pepper, coarsely chopped
2 zucchini, thickly sliced
6 plum tomatoes, coarsely chopped
One 4-ounce can chopped green chilies
2 cups vegetable broth
1 cup chopped fresh cilantro
Tabasco to taste

Preheat the oven to 350°F.

Place the eggplant on a nonstick baking sheet. Bake for 15 to 20 minutes, until lightly browned. Remove from the oven and set aside. While the eggplant is baking, prepare the other vegetables.

Place all the vegetables except the eggplant in a large casserole dish. Mix well. Stir in the chopped green chilies. Pour the vegetable broth over and add ½ cup of the cilantro. Mix well. Cover and bake for 45 minutes. Remove from the oven, stir in the eggplant, return to the oven, and bake for another 30 minutes. Remove from the oven and stir in the remaining cilantro and several dashes of Tabasco, if desired.

Sweet-and-Sour Vegetables

SERVINGS: 4
PREPARATION TIME: 20 MINUTES
COOKING TIME: 15 MINUTES

1 medium onion, coarsely
   chopped
1 green bell pepper,
   coarsely chopped
1 carrot, scrubbed and
   sliced
1 small zucchini, thickly
   sliced
1 cup broccoli florets
1 cup cauliflower florets
One 16-ounce can chopped
   tomatoes

1 cup water
2 tablespoons soy sauce
2 tablespoons rice vinegar
2 tablespoons honey
1½ tablespoons cornstarch
   or arrowroot
1 clove garlic, crushed
½ teaspoon grated fresh
   ginger

Place the onion, green pepper, carrot, zucchini, broccoli, and cauliflower in a large steamer basket. Steam over boiling water until just tender, 5 to 10 minutes. Remove from the heat and place in a serving bowl.

While the vegetables are steaming, combine the tomatoes, the water, and the remaining ingredients in a saucepan. Stir well to dissolve the cornstarch or arrowroot. Bring to a boil, stirring constantly, until the mixture thickens and clears. Pour over the vegetables and toss gently to mix. Serve with potatoes or whole grains.

Savory Baked Vegetables

SERVINGS: 4
PREPARATION TIME: 30 MINUTES
COOKING TIME: 1½ HOURS

4 medium potatoes, scrubbed and sliced
2 carrots, scrubbed and sliced
1 zucchini, thickly sliced
½ pound mushrooms, sliced
1 cup cauliflower florets
1 cup broccoli florets
1 onion, thinly sliced and separated into rings
1½ cups water
2 tablespoons soy sauce
2 cloves garlic, pressed
½ tablespoon paprika

¼ teaspoon curry powder
¼ teaspoon ground cumin
¼ teaspoon dried oregano
⅛ teaspoon dried dill
⅛ teaspoon dried marjoram
⅛ teaspoon freshly ground pepper
Pinch each of ground nutmeg, allspice, cloves, ginger, and coriander
1½ tablespoons cornstarch mixed with ¼ cup cold water

Preheat the oven to 350°F.

Layer the vegetables in a covered casserole dish in the order given. Place the water, soy sauce, garlic, and all the spices in a small jar. Shake to mix well and pour over the vegetables. Cover and bake 1½ hours. Remove from the oven and drain juices into a saucepan. Slowly add the cornstarch and water mixture to the juices in the saucepan. Bring to a boil, stirring constantly, until thickened. Pour the sauce over the vegetables. Serve at once, either by themselves or with whole grains.

Broccoli Mushroom Sauce

SERVINGS: 4 TO 6
PREPARATION TIME: 15 MINUTES
COOKING TIME: 20 MINUTES

2 leeks, washed and sliced
2 cups sliced mushrooms
2 cups broccoli florets
3½ cups water
2 tablespoons soy sauce
1 teaspoon dried oregano

1 teaspoon dried crumbled thyme
½ teaspoon dried crumbled sage
4 tablespoons cornstarch, mixed with ⅓ cup cold water

Sauté the vegetables in ½ cup of the water for 5 minutes. Add the seasonings and the rest of the water. Cook over low heat for 10 minutes. Mix in the cornstarch mixture. Cook and stir until thickened.

Serve over potatoes or grains.

Lo-Cal Stew

SERVINGS: 8
PREPARATION TIME: 20 MINUTES
COOKING TIME: 30 MINUTES

⅓ cup water
1 medium onion, coarsely chopped
1 or 2 cloves garlic, crushed
1 green bell pepper, coarsely chopped
One 28-ounce can chopped tomatoes
4 small zucchini, sliced
2 small yellow crookneck squash, sliced

1 cup sliced green beans
1 cup fresh or frozen corn kernels
1 tablespoon soy sauce
1 tablespoon parsley flakes
1 teaspoon dried basil
1 teaspoon dried oregano
1 tablespoon cornstarch, mixed with ¼ cup cold water

Place the water in a large saucepan with the onion, garlic, and green pepper. Cook and stir until slightly softened, 3 or 4 minutes. Add the tomato, zucchini, squash, and beans. Cover and simmer over medium heat for 15 minutes. Add the corn and seasonings. Cook for another 10 minutes. Add the cornstarch mixture and cook, stirring, until thickened.

Serve with whole grains or potatoes.

Squashy Bean Stew

SERVINGS: 8
PREPARATION TIME: 30 MINUTES
COOKING TIME: 3 HOURS

4 cups water
¾ cup dried pinto beans
¾ cup dried white beans
1 large onion, chopped
1 or 2 cloves garlic, crushed
One 16-ounce can chopped
    tomatoes
1 teaspoon dried basil

1 teaspoon dried oregano
¼ teaspoon crushed red
    pepper flakes
2 cups peeled, chopped
    winter squash
1 cup fresh or frozen
    corn kernels

Place the water and beans in a large soup pot. Bring to a boil, cover, and cook over medium heat for 1½ hours. Add the onion, garlic, tomatoes, and seasonings. Cook for another 30 minutes. Add the squash pieces and cook for 45 minutes longer. Add the corn and cook for another 15 minutes. Serve with whole grains.

Mexican Vegetable Stew

SERVINGS: 4
PREPARATION TIME: 30 MINUTES
COOKING TIME: 30 MINUTES

1 cup water
1 medium onion, chopped
1 clove garlic, minced
1 green bell pepper,
  chopped
1 carrot, chopped
1 stalk celery, chopped
1 zucchini, chopped
1 cup fresh or frozen corn
  kernels

One 16-ounce can kidney
  beans, drained and
  rinsed
1 tablespoon chili powder
½ teaspoon ground cumin
½ teaspoon dried oregano
1 tablespoon cornstarch,
  mixed with ¼ cup cold
  water

Place the water in a medium pot. Add the onion and garlic. Cook and stir for several minutes over medium heat. Add the green pepper, carrot, and celery. Cook, stirring frequently, about 10 minutes. Add the remaining ingredients except the cornstarch mixture. Cover and cook over medium-low heat for 20 minutes, stirring frequently. Stir in the cornstarch mixture and continue to cook, stirring until thickened.

Serve with grains or potatoes.

Garbanzo Stew

SERVINGS: 4
PREPARATION TIME: 15 MINUTES
COOKING TIME: 43 MINUTES

½ cup water
½ cup chopped onion
1 clove garlic, minced
1 cup chopped tomato
¼ teaspoon paprika
¼ teaspoon dried oregano
⅛ teaspoon freshly ground
   pepper
Dash Tabasco

1 cup cooked garbanzo
   beans, drained and
   rinsed
½ cup chopped winter
   squash
One 6-ounce can spicy
   tomato juice
1 cup fresh spinach,
   washed and chopped

Place the water, onion, and garlic in a large pot. Cook, stirring occasionally, until the onion is softened slightly, about 5 minutes. Add the tomato and seasonings. Cook for 5 more minutes. Add the garbanzo beans, squash, and tomato juice. Cover and cook for 30 minutes. Stir in the spinach and cook until softened, 2 to 3 minutes.

Alu Gobi
(Potato Cauliflower Curry)

SERVINGS: 6
PREPARATION TIME: 20 MINUTES
COOKING TIME: 35 MINUTES

1 medium onion,
chopped
1 to 1½ cups water
1 tablespoon ground
cumin
1 tablespoon ground
ginger
1 tablespoon ground
turmeric
½ tablespoon chili
powder

1 head cauliflower, cut
into florets
2 white potatoes,
peeled and cubed
1 or 2 tablespoons soy
sauce
Chopped fresh
cilantro for garnish

Place the onion and water in a large saucepan. Cook, stirring, until the onion is tender. Add the spices, stirring several times, and add the cauliflower and potatoes and another ½ cup water. Cook, covered, over low heat until the vegetables are tender, 25 to 30 minutes. Check occasionally and add more water if necessary to keep the vegetables from sticking to the pan. Before serving, stir in soy sauce to taste and garnish with cilantro.

Curried Eggplant

SERVINGS: 4

PREPARATION TIME: 20 MINUTES

COOKING TIME: EGGPLANT 45 MINUTES, CURRY 20 TO 25 MINUTES

1 large eggplant
½ cup water
1 medium onion, chopped
1 tablespoon grated fresh
ginger
½ teaspoon cumin seeds
1 green bell pepper,
chopped
1 tomato, peeled and
chopped (see Note)

2 teaspoons ground
coriander
1 teaspoon ground turmeric
1 teaspoon ground cumin
1 teaspoon paprika
¼ teaspoon freshly ground
pepper
1 tablespoon soy sauce
½ cup chopped fresh
cilantro

Preheat the oven to 400°F.

Prick the eggplant all over with a fork. Place in a shallow baking dish and bake until very soft, about 45 minutes. Remove from the oven and cool. Cut in half and scoop out the pulp. Chop the pulp and set aside.

Place ¼ cup of the water in a saucepan. Add the onion, ginger, and cumin seeds. Cook, stirring occasionally, until the onion softens slightly. Add the green pepper, tomato, coriander, turmeric, cumin, paprika, and pepper. Cook, stirring occasionally, for 5 minutes. Add the remaining water and soy sauce. Cook for another 5 minutes. Stir in the eggplant and cook for 5 minutes longer. Add the cilantro, stir several times, and remove from the heat.

Note: To peel the tomato, plunge it into boiling water, then remove it and slip off the skin.

Mattar Guchi
(Indian Spiced Peas and Mushrooms)

SERVINGS: 4
PREPARATION TIME: 15 MINUTES
COOKING TIME: 20 MINUTES

⅓ cup water
1 small onion, finely chopped
1 garlic clove, minced
½ to 1 teaspoon curry powder
½ teaspoon ground cumin
¼ teaspoon ground coriander
⅛ teaspoon ground cinnamon
Pinch ground cloves
½ pound mushrooms, sliced

One 15½-ounce can chopped tomatoes with their juice
One 10-ounce box frozen peas, thawed
One 8-ounce can garbanzo beans, drained and rinsed
Chopped fresh cilantro and freshly ground pepper for garnish

Place the water in a large pot. Add the onion and garlic and cook, stirring until the onion softens slightly. Add all the spices and cook 1 minute. Add the remaining ingredients except the pepper and cilantro. Simmer over low heat for 15 minutes.

Serve over rice or potatoes, garnished with cilantro and pepper, if desired.

APPENDIX

Additional Recipes That Fit Your Weight-Loss Program

Recipes from the previous McDougall books that fit the principles of the McDougall Program for Maximum Weight Loss are listed below. An asterisk (*) indicates the recipe fits the very low-calorie green and yellow vegetable category.

McDougall Books with Recipes:

The McDougall Plan (New Win Publishing, 1983)

The McDougall Health-Supporting Cookbook, Volume I (New Win Publishing, 1985)

The McDougall Health-Supporting Cookbook, Volume II (New Win Publishing, 1986)

The McDougall Program: 12 Days to Dynamic Health (Plume, 1991)

The New McDougall Cookbook (Dutton, 1993)

These books can be found in most bookstores or can be ordered by calling (707) 576-1654 or writing P.O. Box 14039, Santa Rosa, CA 95402.

Recipes from *The McDougall Plan*

Apple Butter
Baked Stuffed Squash
Barbequed Beans
Barley and Beans
Barley-Mushroom Soup
Brazilian Black Beans with
  Marinated Tomatoes
Brown Rice
Butch's Chili
Chili
Chinese Vegetable Sauce
Curried Beans
Dal
Easy Curried Lentil or Pea
  Soup
Easy Ratatouille*
Eggplant Dip*
Enchilada Sauce
Fried Rice
Garbanzo Puree
Golden Potatoes
Hearty Brown Stew
Heather's Mushroom Delight
Hot German Potato Salad
Hot Mexican Salsa
Ketchup Sauce
Latin Black Bean Soup
Layered Dinner
Lemon-Garlic Dressing
Lentil Soup
Marinara Spaghetti Sauce
Middle East Vegetable Stew
Mild Gazpacho*
Mixed Sprout Salad
Mushroom Gravy
Onion Soup*
Paella

Patrick's Simple Refried Beans
Pea Soup
Peasant's Pie
Pizza Sauce
Potato Bhaji
Potato Scramble
Rice Summer Salad
Sherried Rice
Shish-Kebabs*
Simple Tomato Pasta Sauce
Sloppy Lentils
Spanish Bulgur
Spanish Rice
Spicy Gravy
Spicy Mexican Topping
Spicy Vegetable Stew
Stove-Top Stew
Stuffed Cabbage Rolls
Stuffed Peppers
Sweet and Sour Lentil Soup
Sweet and Sour Lentil Stew
Szechuan Eggplant*
Tabouli
Taco Beans
Thick French Tomato Dressing
Tomato Scalloped Potatoes
Tomato-Onion Soup
Tossed Green Rice
Vegetable Chop Suey
Vegetable Curry
Vegetable Soup
Vegetable Stew
Vegetables and Rice
Vegetable-Bean Soup
Vegetable-Stuffed Peppers with
  Spicy Tomato Sauce
White Bean Soup

Recipes from *The McDougall Health-Supporting Cookbook*, Volume I

Ann's garbanzo casserole
Autumn barley stew
Azuki rice
Baked vegetables
Baked limas with tomato sauce
Baked potatoes
Banana freeze
Barley soup
Barley lentil surprise
Barley-mushroom casserole
Bean mixtures
Black bean soup
Black-eyed peas
Boiled dinner
Broiled zucchini*
Butch's bean soup
Calico soup
Caponata
Carob fruit fondue
Cauliflower curry*
Celeste's salsa
Chinese cabbage and bean
   sprouts*
Chinese hot salad*
Chinese peas and mushrooms*
Chunky vegetable sauce
Colorful mashed potatoes
Corn & potato soup
Country vegetables*
Creamy potato sauce
Curried lentils & rice
Curried garbanzos
Curried vegetable stew
Curried pea soup
Curry sauce
Dilly vegetables*
Dinner millet
Dried mushroom & vegetable
   saute*
Easy split moong dal

Elaine's spicy lentils
Flake casserole
French tomato dressing
Fruit salad
Garam-masala (Indian curry
   spice mix)
Garbanzo stew
Garden soup
Gazpacho*
Ginger sauce
Golden sauce
Grain soup
Grain pilaf
Grainy vegetable soup
Herbed vinegar dressing
Herbed green beans*
Homemade chili dip
Hot yammy soup
Indian cabbage*
Indian vegetables
Indian pulao
Indonesian fried rice
Italian green beans*
Jan's Jamaican pumpkin soup
Judy's navy bean soup
Ketchup
Layered rice casserole
Lee's cabbage salad*
Leftovers soup
Lemon sauce
Lentil dahl
Lentil soup II
Lentil-vegetable soup
Lentil-rice burgers
Lima bean jambalaya
Lima bean spinach
Mashed potatoes
Mexican zucchini*
Millet stew
Molded gazpacho salad*

Mung bean sprout salad*
Mushroom curry
New potato salad
Onion-mushroom sauce
Orange soup
Oriental spice gravy
Oriental tomato sauce
Oriental vegetables*
Polynesian vegetables
Potato soup
Potato casserole
Potato and cauliflower curry
Quick tomato-rice soup
Quick enchilada sauce
Quick confetti rice
Quick beet soup*
Quick brown stew
Quintabean soup
Ratatouille*
Raw vegetable platter*
Refried beans
Rice-mushroom casserole
Russian dressing
Saffron brown rice
Savory brown rice
Seven bean soup
Shredded salad*
Simple baked eggplant*
Simple pea soup
Slow-cooked dried beans
Southern black beans
Spaghetti sauce

Spaghetti squash surprise*
Spicy green beans*
Spinach salad*
Spinach rice casserole
Split pea curry
Sprout salad
Sprouted lettuce salad
Squash dinner pie
Steamed vegetables with gravy
Stove-top zucchini casserole
Sweet potato soup
Sweet squash pie
Sweet-sour vegetable saute
Szechuan sauce
Szechuan shish kebabs*
Tamari sauce
Tomato soup*
Tomato-onion-cucumber salad*
Tossed salad*
Twice-baked potatoes
Vegetable stock
Vegetable melange*
Vegetable salad provencale*
Vegie salad dressing
Vichyssoise
Vinegar dressing
White bean & vegetable soup
Wicked mushrooms
Wilted lettuce
Yam 'n' apple casserole
Zesty peppers*
Zucchini corn casserole*

Recipes from *The McDougall Health-Supporting Cookbook*, Volume II

African millet and beans
Ann's super curry
Baked millet supreme
Baked potato salad
Bamboo steamed fresh
  vegetables

Barbecued burgers
Barley vegetable casserole
Basil bean soup
Bean and vegetable casserole
Black bean chili
Black beans and nectarines

Broiled Dijon tomatoes
Buddha's delight
Cajun bean stew
Cajun potatoes
Cajun spices
Carrot soup
Chinese spicy vegetables*
Chinese vegetables
Christmas Eve soup*
Colcannon
Cold brown rice salad
Colorful coleslaw
Country vegetable soup
Cream of broccoli soup*
Crispy yam treat
Deviled green beans*
Dilly stuffed cabbage
Fassolada
Fejoiada
Flavorful "refried" beans
French peasant soup
French vegetable soup
Fresh vegetable chili
Fresh vegetable soup
Garbanzo salad
Ginger carrots
Grainy vegetable stew
Greek stew
Green bean special*
Green bulgur
Green onion soup
Haposai
Hearty potato vegetable curry
Hearty vegetable soup
Hunter's flat bean soup
India eggplant*
Israeli wheat berry stew
Italian cauliflower*
Italian potato casserole
Janine's spaghetti sauce
Japanese soup stock
Kidney bean spread
Korean rice and potatoes

Lemon broccoli*
Lentil salad
Lentil-mushroom pate
Lima bean salad
Luau rice
Mandarin eggplant
Marinated cucumbers
Marinated mushrooms
Marinated onions*
Mashed stuffed squash
Mexican bean soup
Mexican bulgur
Mexican corn
Mexican gazpacho*
Mexican rice
Moroccan garbanzo soup
Moroccan stew
Multi grain stew
Multiple bean casserole
Mungo beans
Mushroom soup
New Orleans Creole sauce
Nine staples soup
North African bean soup
Oriental dipping sauce
Pea and potato curry
Poi stew
Popcorn
Potato and bean soup
Potato chowder
Potato-onion bake
Potato-veggie dinner
Potatoes with dill
Quick chili
Quick Oriental cabbage*
Quick rice dinner
Quick saucy vegetables
Rice and corn salad
Roasted legumes
Russian borscht
Salsa cruda
Saucy Brussels sprouts*
Seven layer casserole

Sherried tomato soup
Sherrie's oil-free dressing
Simple vegetable soup
Six-way-fun chili
South American bean stew
South of the border soup
Southern style black eyed peas
Spanish garbanzo soup
Spicy bean spread
Spicy bean spread II
Spicy Chinese rice
Spicy lentil filling
Spicy Mexican tomato sauce
Spicy mixed bean chili
Spicy pea soup
Spicy vegetable sauce
Summer stew
Summer vegetable delight

Super sprout salad
Sushi
Syrian potato salad
Three bean salad
Tomato relish
Umeboshi plum stew
Unforgettable Chinese
   eggplant*
Vegetable salad
Vegetable spaghetti sauce
Vegetables a la grecque
White bean spread
Wild rice casserole
Wild rice soup
Winter grains soup
Zucchini casserole*
Zucchini velvet soup
Zucchini-potato curry

Recipes from *The McDougall Program: Twelve Days to Dynamic Health*

American Vegetable Stew
Baked Apple
Baked Potato Salad
Baked Winter Squash with Five-
   Grain, Brown, and Wild Rice
   Holiday Stuffing
Black-eyed peas for Cajun Sauce
Breakfast Rice with Fruit
Cajun Rice
Cajun Sauce
California Stew
Cucumber Vinaigrette Salad
Curried Vegetables
Double Rice and Greens
French Market Soup
Frozen Hash-Brown Potatoes
Garbanzo Bean Spread
Gingered Vegetable Soup
Kidney Bean Spread
Lentil Stew

Lima Bean Curry
Marinara Sauce
Mexican Corn on the Cob
Mexican Vegetable Sauce
Microwaved Apple Wedges
Microwaved Baked Potato with
   All the Toppings
Mixed Bean Salad
Picante Black Beans
Potato Scramble
Quick Broiled Zucchini*
Quick "Fried" Potatoes
Quick Garbanzo Bean Soup
Quick Oatmeal
Quick Saucy Vegetables
Red and White Salad*
Rice Cakes and Jam
Saucy Cauliflower*
Savory Baked Beans
Seasoned Potatoes

Sliced Tomatoes with Salsa
Sparkling Minted Fruit
Special Stuffed Peppers
Spicy Bean Spread
Spicy Chili Beans
Spicy Pinto Bean Spread
Split Green Pea Soup

Split Green Pea and Vegetable
  Stew
Stuffed Tomato Salad
Sweet and Sour Vegetables
Sweet and Spicy Garbanzo
  Stew
White Bean Spread

Recipes from *The New McDougall Cookbook*

Adas Bi Sabaanikh (Lentil and
  Spinach Soup)
Baked Potato Skins
Barbecued Onions
Barley Salad
Bean Burgers
Bean and Rice Salad
Better Than Firesign Potatoes
Black Bean and Corn Salad
Black Bean Soup with Cilantro
  and Orange
Borscht
Broccoli Barley Toss
Broccoli Garbanzo Stew
Broccomole*
Brussels Sprouts with Creamy
  Horseradish Sauce
Bulghur-stuffed Peppers
Cajun Black-eyed Pea Stew
Cajun Spices
Cajun Vegetable Sauce
Cauliflower Potato Curry
Chili-Cilantro Dressing
Chunky Enchilada Sauce
Chunky Gazpacho*
Chunky Vegetable Marinara
  Sauce
Cilantro, Chutney
Confetti Beans
Couscous Salad
Creamy White Bean Soup
Cuban Black Beans

Cucumber Dill Crunch*
Curried Bean Sandwich
  Spread
Curried Red Lentil Soup
Curried Rice Salad
Drunken Bean Soup
Dry Soup
Dutch Vegetable Whip
East-West Breakfast
Eggplant and Garbanzo Stew
Eggplant Spread*
Extra-spicy Lentil Chili
Five-grain Medley
Fresh Salsa
Fresh Tomato Sauce
  with Garlic
Garam Masala
Garbanzo Broccoli Stew
Garlic Soup
Golden Potato Wedges
Golden Spicy Cauliflower
Grandma Gibson's Split Pea
  Soup
Grated Potato Bake
Green Bean Medley*
Green Bean Soup*
Green Chili Sauce
Green Enchilada Sauce
Green Papaya Salad*
Green Pepper and Tomato
  Teriyaki
Harvest Vegetable Sauté

Hash-brown Medley
Hearty Brown Stew
Hearty Vegetable Broth
Indian Garbanzo and Tomato Stew
Indian Lentil Sandwich Spread
Jiffy Vegetarian Posole
Layered Vegetable Casserole
Lentil Patties
Lentil Tomato Soup
Light Vegetable Broth
Lima Bean Soup
Marinara Sauce
Marinated Lentil Salad
Mashed Potatoes
Mexican Rice
Millet Loaf
Mixed Bean and Vegetable Soup
Moroccan Chick-peas
Multigrain Hot Cereal
Mustard Squash*
Oats and Millet
Okra Gumbo
Peperonata
Potato Curry
Potato Kugel
Potato-Leek Soup
Quick-sautéed Spiced Vegetables with Rice
Quinoa Salad
Ratatouille*
Red and Green Salad
Red-Hot Chili
Red Pepper Sauce
Roasted Garlic Spread
Sandwich Cheese
Sautéed Italian Zucchini*
Savory Lentils
Savory Salad Dressing
Seasoned Oven Fries
Shiitake Mushroom Sauce

Smashed Beans
Southwestern Black Bean Soup
Spaghetti Squash Marinara
Spanish Rice
Spanish-Style Vegetable Casserole
Spicy Black Bean Chili
Spicy Carrot Soup
Spicy Garbanzo Bean Soup
Spicy Mexican Bean Salad
Spicy Mixed Bean Soup
Spicy Pasta Sauce
Spicy Potato Chunks
Spicy Red Beans
Spicy Rice and Beans
Spicy Three-Bean Salad
Spicy Vegetable Stew
Spicy Yam Stew
Spinach-Mushroom Soup
Split Pea Soup with Lentils and Vegetables
Spring Salad
Stuffed Collard Greens
Sunshine Texas Crude
Sweet-potato Puffs
Sweet Squash Soup
Szechwan Sauce
Tabouli
Tangy Mushroom Sauce
Tasty Blender Salsa*
Texas Crude
Texas-style Black-eyed Pea Soup
Thai Cabbage Salad*
Three Bean Chili
Three Bean Pilaf
Three-grain Medley
Tomato Rice Salad
Tomato Salad*
Twin Sisters Vegetable Soup
Two Bean and Rice Salad
Two Bean Pasta Sauce

Vegetable-Barley Salad
Vegetables Provençale*
Vegetarian Paella
White Bean Salad

Yellow-pepper Sauce
Zesty Red Potato Salad
Zucchini and Eggplant Stuffed
   Tomatoes

REFERENCES

Chapter 1

Carl Lewis on the McDougall Program:
 Marx, J. Catching up with the world's fastest human. *Runner's World* August
  1992, pages 62–69.

Quote: cancer easier to cure than obesity:
 Council on Scientific Affairs. Treatment of obesity in adults. *JAMA*
  260:2547, 1988.

Chapter 2

After starving, people will eat to the point of death:
 Keys, A. et al. *The Biology of Human Starvation.* Minneapolis, University of
  Minnesota Press, 1950, page 1385.

Dieting leads to changes that make weight regain easier:
 Polivy, J. Dieting and binging. *Am Psychologist* 40:193, 1985.
 Frankle, R. *Obesity and Weight Control.* The Health Professionals Guide to
  Understanding and Treatment. Rockville, MD: Aspen, 1988. Page 99.
 Manore, M. Energy expenditure at rest and during exercise in nonobese
  female dieters and in nondieting control subjects. *Am J Clin Nutr* 54:41,
  1991.
 Blackburn, G. Weight cycling: the experience of human dieters. *Am J Clin
  Nutr* 49:1105, 1989.

Steen, S. Metabolic effects of repeated weight loss and regain in adolescent wrestlers. *JAMA* 260:47, 1988.

Dulloo, A. Adaptive changes in energy expenditure during refeeding following low-calorie intake: evidence for a specific metabolic component favoring fat storage. *Am J Clin Nutr* 52:415, 1990.

Kern, P. The effects of weight loss on the activity and expression of adipose-tissue lipoprotein lipase in very obese humans. *N Engl J Med* 322:1053, 1990.

Fat provides no satisfaction/carbohydrate satisfies hunger:

Blundell, J. Dietary fat and the control of energy intake: evaluating the effects of fat on meal size and postmeal satiety. *Am J Clin Nutr* 57 (suppl): 772S, 1993.

Tremblay, A. Impact of dietary fat content and fat oxidation on energy intake in humans. *Am J Clin Nutr* 49:799, 1989.

Flatt, J. Dietary fat, carbohydrate balance, and weight maintenance: effects of exercise. *Am J Clin Nutr* 45:296, 1987.

Chapter 3

Your hunger drive demands you consume sufficient carbohydrates:

Blundell, J. Dietary fat and the control of energy intake: evaluating the effects of fat on meal size and postmeal satiety. *Am J Clin Nutr* 57 (suppl): 772S, 1993.

Ravussin, E. Pathophysiology of obesity. *Lancet* 340:404, 1992.

Duncan, K. The effects of high and low energy density diets on satiety, energy intake, and eating time of obese and nonobese subjects. *Am J Clin Nutr* 37:763: 1983.

Miller, W. Diet composition, energy intake, and exercise in relation to body fat in men and women. *Am J Clin Nutr* 52:426, 1990.

Protein encourages aggressive behavior/Carbohydrate quiets irritability and depression:

Wurtman, J. Carbohydrate craving in obese people: suppression by treatments affecting serotoninergic transmission. *Int J Eating Disorders* 1:2, 1981.

Wurtman, J. Effect of nutrient intake on premenstrual depression. *Am J Obstet Gynecol* 161:1228, 1989.

Wurtman J. Behavioural effects of nutrients. *Lancet* 1:1145, 1983.

Glaeser, B. Changes in brain levels of acidic, basic, and neutral amino acids after consumption of single meals containing various portions of protein. *J Neurochem* 41:1016, 1983.

Lieberman, H. The effects of dietary neurotransmitter precursors on human behavior. *Am J Clin Nutr* 42:366, 1985.

Chapter 4

Cost of storing fat is 3 percent of calories:
Danfourth, E. Diet and obesity. *Am J Clin Nutr* 41:1132, 1985.

The fat you eat is the fat you wear (same chemical structure):
Leo, T. Hydrogenated oils and fats: the presence of chemically-modified fatty acids in human adipose tissue. *Am J Clin Nutr* 34:877, 1981.
London, S. Fatty acid composition of subcutaneous adipose tissue and diet in postmenopausal US women. *Am J Clin Nutr* 54:340, 1991.
Insull, W. Studies of arteriosclerosis in Japanese and American men. I. Comparison of fatty acid composition of adipose tissue. *J Clin Invest* 48:1313, 1969.
Dayton, S. Composition of lipids in human serum and adipose tissues during prolonged feeding of a diet high in unsaturated fats. *J Lipid Res* 7:103, 1966.
Hirsch, J. Studies of adipose tissues in man. A microtechnique for sampling and analysis. *Am J Clin Nutr* 8:499, 1960.
Beynen, A. A mathematical relationship between the fatty acid composition of the diet and that of the adipose tissue in man. *Am J Clin Nutr* 33:81, 1980.

Carbohydrates don't turn to fat under usual conditions:
Oliver, O. Oxidative and nonoxidative macronutrient disposal in lean and obese subjects after mixed meals. *Am J Clin Nutr* 55:630, 1992.
Acheson, K. Carbohydrate metabolism and de novo lipogenesis in human obesity. *Am J Clin Nutr* 45:78, 1987.
Hellerstein, M. Measurement of de novo hepatic lipogenesis in humans using stable isotopes. *J Clin Invest* 87:1841, 1991.
Acheson, K. Glycogen storage capacity and de novo lipogenesis during massive carbohydrate overfeeding in man. *Am J Clin Nutr* 48: 240, 1988.

Chapter 5

Hunger satisfaction begins with chewing:
Smith, G. Peripheral control of appetite. *Lancet* 2:88, 1983.
Duncan, K. The effects of high and low energy density diets on satiety, energy intake, and eating time of obese and nonobese subjects. *Am J Clin Nutr* 37:763, 1983.

Bulk alone fills the stomach:
Smith, M. The role of bulk in the control of eating. *J Comp Physiology Psychology* 55:115, 1962.

Fiber blocks fat absorption:
   Isaksson, N. Effects of dietary fiber on pancreatic enzyme activities of ile-
      ostomy evacuates and on excretion of fat and nitrogen in the rat. *Scand
      J Gastroenterol* 18:417, 1983.
   Sandberg, A. The effect of citrus pectin on the absorption of nutrients in
      the small intestine. *Hum Nutr* 37C:171, 1983.

Insulin keeps the fat in fat cells:
   Cahill, G. Hormone-fuel interrelationships during fasting. *J Clin Invest*
      45:1751, 1966.
   Eckel, R. Insulin resistance: an adaption for weight maintenance. *Lancet* 340:
      1452, 1990.

Most obese people have elevated insulin:
   Karam, J. Excessive insulin response to glucose in obese subjects as mea-
      sured by immunochemical assay. *Diabetes* 12:197, 1963.

Weight loss lowers insulin:
   Farrant, P. Insulin release in response to oral glucose in obesity: The effect
      of reduction of body weight. *Diabetologia* 5:198, 1969.

Insulin shots and diabetic pills encourage weight gain:
   Welle, S. Effect of a sulfonylurea and insulin on energy expenditure in type
      II diabetes mellitus. *J Clin Endocrinol Metab* 66:593, 1988.
   Harris, M. Exogenous insulin therapy slows weight loss in type 2 diabetic
      patients. *Int J Obes* 12:149, 1988.

Chapter 6

Processing of grains means greater absorption of calories and higher insulin:
   Jenkins, D. Wholemeal versus wholegrain breads: proportion of whole or
      cracked grain and the glycemic index. *Br Med J* 297:958, 1988.
   O'Dea, K. Physical factors influencing postprandial glucose and insulin re-
      sponses to starch. *Am J Clin Nutr* 33:760, 1980.
   O'Dea, K. The rate of starch hydrolysis in vitro as a predictor of metabolic
      responses to complex carbohydrates in vivo. *Am J Clin Nutr* 34:1991,
      1981.
   Snow, P. Factors affecting the rate of hydrolysis of starch in food. *Am J Clin
      Nutr* 34:2721, 1981.

Legumes slow absorption and reduce insulin and glucose response:
   Thorne, M. Factors affecting starch digestibility and the glycemic response
      with special reference to legumes. *Am J Clin Nutr* 38:481, 1983.
   O'Dea, K. The rate of starch hydrolysis in vitro does not predict the meta-
      bolic responses of legumes in vivo. *Am J Clin Nutr* 38:382, 1983.
   Würsch, P. Metabolic effects of instant beans and potato over 6 hours. *Am
      J Clin Nutr* 48:1418, 1988.

Jenkins, D. Effect of processing on digestibility and the blood glucose response: a study of lentils. *Am J Clin Nutr* 36:1093, 1982.

Lin, H. Sustained slowing effect of lentils on gastric emptying of solids in humans and dogs. *Gastroenterology* 102:787, 1992.

Cooking increases blood sugar and insulin responses:

Collings, P. Effect of cooking on serum glucose and insulin responses to starch. *Br Med J* 282:1032, 1981.

Douglass, J. Raw diet and insulin requirement. *Ann Intern Med* 82:61, 1975.

Horowitz, D. Raw diet and diabetes mellitus. *Ann Intern Med* 82:853, 1975.

Douglass, J. Effects of a raw food diet on hypertension and obesity. *South Med J* 78:841, 1985.

Processing fruit increases insulin and blood sugar responses:

Haber, G. Depletion and disruption of dietary fiber. Effects on satiety, plasma-glucose, and serum-insulin. *Lancet* 2:679, 1977.

Fruit raises insulin:

Roongpisuthipong, C. Postprandial glucose and insulin responses to various tropical fruits of equivalent carbohydrate content in non-insulin dependent diabetes mellitus. *Diabetes Res Clin Pract* 14:123, 1991.

Fruit (fructose) raises triglycerides more than do other sugars:

Hallfrisch, J. Metabolic effects of dietary fructose. *Faseb J* 4:2652, 1990.

Sugar raises insulin and blood sugar more than does starch:

Reiser, S. Isocaloric exchange of dietary starch and sucrose in humans. II. Effect on fasting blood insulin, glucose, and glucagon and on insulin and glucose response to a sucrose load. *Am J Clin Nutr* 32:2206, 1979.

Small amounts of sugar are of little consequence:

Bantle, J. Postprandial glucose and insulin responses to meals containing different carbohydrates in normal and diabetic subjects. *N Engl J Med* 309:7, 1983.

Eating fat with sugar is worse:

Suzuki, M. Simultaneous ingestion of fat and sucrose may contribute to development of obesity: a larger body fat accumulation as compared with their separate ingestion. *Fed Proc* 45:481, 1986.

Sclafani, A. Dietary-induced overeating. *Ann NY Acad Sci* 575:281, 1989.

Obese people tend to gorge:

Adams, C. Periodicity of eating: implications for human consumption. *Nutr Res* 1:525, 1981.

Southgate, D. Nibblers, gorgers, snackers, and grazers. Eating little and (very) often is beneficial to health. *Br Med J* 300:136, 1990.

Frequent meals reduce blood glucose and insulin response:
Bertelsen, J. Effect of meal frequency on blood glucose, insulin, and free fatty acids in NIDDM subjects. *Diabetes Care* 16:4, 1993.
Jenkins, D. Nibbling versus gorging: metabolic advantages of increased meal frequency. *N Engl J Med* 321:929, 1989.

Thinking of eating may burn calories (cephalic thermogenesis):
Allard, M. Effects of cold acclimation, cold exposure, and palatability on postprandial thermogenesis in rats. *Int J Obesity* 12:169, 1987.
LeBlanc, J. Effect of meal size and frequency on the postprandial thermogenesis of dogs. *Am J Physiol* 250:E144, 1986.
Brand, J. Chemical senses in the release of gastric and pancreatic secretions. *Ann Rev Nutr* 2:249, 1982.

Chew foods thoroughly for satisfaction:
Duncan, K. The effects of high and low energy density diets on satiety, energy intake, and eating time of obese and nonobese subjects. *Am J Clin Nutr* 37:763: 1983.

Restricting variety of foods decreases intake:
Spiegel, T. Effects of variety on food intake of underweight, normal-weight and overweight women. *Appetite* 15:47, 1990.
Rolls, B. Pleasantness changes and food intake in a varied four-course meal. *Appetite* 5:337, 1984.
Rolls, B. Variety in a meal enhances food intake in man. *Physiol Behav* 26:215, 1981.
Bellisle, F. The structure of meals in humans: eating and drinking patterns in lean and obese subjects. *Physiol Behav* 27:649, 1981.

Complete nutrients from simple starches:
Lopez de Romana, G. Prolonged consumption of potato-based diets by infants and small children. *J Nutr* 111:1430, 1981.
Lopez de Romana, G. Utilization of the protein and energy of the white potato by human infants. *J Nutr* 110:1849, 1980.
Kon, S. The value of whole potatoes in human nutrition. *Biochemical J* 22:258, 1928.

Kempner: a simple, safe solution to massive obesity:
Kempner, W. Treatment of massive obesity with Rice/Reduction Diet Program. *Arch Intern Med* 135:1575, 1975.

Fiber decreases insulin response:
Albrink, M. Effect of high- and low-fiber diets on plasma lipids and insulin. *Am J Clin Nutr* 32:1486, 1979.
Potter, J. Effect of test meals of varying dietary fiber content on plasma insulin and glucose response. *Am J Clin Nutr* 34:328, 1981.

Salt and obesity:
  Thorburn, A. Salt and glycaemic response. *Br Med J* 292:1697, 1986.
  O'Donnell, L. Failure of salt to increase starch digestibility and glycemic response. *Br Med J* 296:394, 1988.

Hot red peppers increase calorie expenditure:
  Cameron-Smith, D. Capsaicin and dihydrocapsaicin stimulate oxygen consumption in the perfused rat hindlimb. *Int J Obes* 14:259, 1990.

Artificial sweeteners may slow weight loss:
  Rogers, P. Uncoupling sweet taste and calories: comparison of the effects of glucose and three intense sweeteners on hunger and food intake. *Physiol Behav* 43:547, 1988.
  Tordoff, M. How do non-nutritive sweeteners increase food intake? *Appetite* 11(suppl):5, 1988.
  Brala, P. Effects of sweetness perception and caloric value of a preload on short term intake. *Physiol Behav* 30:1, 1983.
  Ionescu, E. Taste-induced changes in plasma insulin and glucose turnover in lean and obese rats. *Diabetes* 37:773, 1988.
  Wurtman, R. Neurochemical changes following high-dose aspartame with dietary carbohydrates. *N Engl J Med* (letter) 309:429, 1983.
  Tordoff, M. Oral stimulation with aspartame increases hunger. *Physiol Behav* 47:555, 1990.
  Blundell, J. Paradoxical effects of an intense sweetener (Aspartame) on appetite. *Lancet* (letter) 1:1092, 1986.

Water causes food to enter intestine faster:
  Cooke, A. Control of gastric emptying and motility. *Gastroenterology* 68:804, 1975.
  Schusdziarra, V. Effect of solid and liquid carbohydrates upon postprandial pancreatic endocrine function. *J Clin Endocrinol Metab* 53:16, 1981.

Chapter 7

Progesterone increases appetite:
  Landau, R. The appetite of pregnant women. *JAMA* 250:3323, 1983.

No increase in food intake in pregnant women in rural countries:
  Tuazon, M. Energy requirements of pregnancy in the Philippines. *Lancet* 2:1129, 1987.
  Durnin, J. Is nutritional status endangered by virtually no extra intake during pregnancy? *Lancet* 2:823, 1985.
  Lawrence, M. Maintenance energy cost of pregnancy in rural Gambian women and the influence of dietary status. *Lancet* 2:363, 1984.

Women carry 20 percent extra weight effortlessly:
  Jones, C. Fatness and the energy cost of carrying loads in African women.
    Lancet (letter) 2:1331, 1987.

Small women need 1,000 calories a day for basic metabolism:
  Cunningham, J. A reanalysis of the factors influencing basal metabolic rate
    in normal adults. *Am J Clin Nutr* 33:2372, 1980.
  Cunningham, J. Body composition and resting metabolic rate: the myth of
    feminine metabolism. *Am J Clin Nutr* 36:721, 1982.

Fat distribution and sex hormones:
  Steingrimsdottir, L. Hormonal modulation of adipose tissue lipoprotein lip-
    ase may alter food intake in rats. *Am J Physiol* 239:E162, 1980.
  Evans, D. Relationship of androgenic activity to body fat topography, fat
    cell morphology, and metabolic aberrations in premenopausal women.
    J Clin Endocrinol Metab 57:304, 1983.

Fat men with higher risk factors:
  Kalkhoff, R. Relationship of body fat distribution to blood pressure, car-
    bohydrate tolerance, and plasma lipids in healthy obese women. *J Lab
    Clin Med* 102:621, 1983.
  Krotkiewski, M. Impact of obesity on metabolism in men and women. Im-
    portance of regional adipose tissue distribution. *J Clin Invest* 72:1150,
    1983.

Chapter 8

Obese people underreport food intake:
  Lightman, S. Discrepancy between self-reported and actual caloric intake
    and exercise in obese subjects. *N Engl J Med* 327:1893, 1992.
  Bandini, L. Validity of reported energy intake in obese and nonobese ado-
    lescents. *Am J Clin Nutr* 52:421, 1990.

Obese people are found to eat less food:
  Thompson, J. Exercise and obesity: etiology, physiology, and intervention.
    Psych Bull 91:55, 1982.
  Maxfield, E. Patterns of food intake and physical activity in obesity. *J Am
    Diet Assoc* 49:406, 1966.
  Beaudoin, R. Food intakes of obese and nonobese women. *J Am Diet Assoc*
    29:29, 1953.
  McCarthy, M. Dietary and activity patterns of obese women in Trinidad.
    J Am Diet Assoc 48:33, 1966.
  Hutson, E. Measures of body fat and related factors in normal adults. *J Am
    Diet Assoc* 47:179, 1965.
  Bradfield, R. Energy expenditure and heart rate of obese high school girls.
    Am J Clin Nutr 24:1482, 1971.

Stefanik, P. Caloric intake in relation to energy output of obese and non-obese adolescent boys. *Am J Clin Nutr* 7:55, 1959.

Johnson, M. Relative importance of inactivity and overeating in the energy balance of obese high school girls. *Am J Clin Nutr* 4:37, 1956.

Hampton, M. Caloric and nutrient intakes of teenagers. *J Am Diet Assoc* 50:385, 1967.

Gazzaniga, J. Relationship between diet composition and body fatness, with adjustment for resting energy expenditure and physical activity, in pre-adolescent children. *Am J Clin Nutr* 58:21, 1993.

Obese people burn fewer calories:
Jequier, E. New evidence for a thermogenic defect in human obesity. *Int J Obesity* 9(suppl):1, 1985.

Even after weight loss, obese people are still metabolically efficient:
Froidevaux, F. Energy expenditure in obese women before and during weight loss, after refeeding, and in the weight-relapse period. *Am J Clin Nutr* 57:35, 1993.

Kern, P. The effects of weight loss on the activity and expression of adipose-tissue lipoprotein lipase in very obese humans. *N Engl J Med* 322:1053, 1990.

Obese girls exercised less:
Johnson, M. Relative importance of inactivity and overeating in the energy balance of obese high school girls. *Am J Clin Nutr* 4:37, 1956.

Too many fat cells:
Salans, L. Studies of human adipose tissue. Adipose cell size and number in nonobese and obese people. *J Clin Invest* 52:929, 1973.

Brook, C. Relation between age of onset of obesity and size and number of adipose cells. *Br Med J* 2:25, 1972.

Björntorp, P. Effects of refeeding on adipocyte metabolism in the rat. *Int J Obesity* 4:11, 1980.

Obesity in pets and their owners:
Mason, E. Obesity in pet dogs. *Veterinary Record* 86:612, 1970.

Quotes on obesity:
Van Itallie, T. Bad news and good news about obesity. *N Engl J Med* 314:239, 1986.

Garrow, J. Predisposition to obesity. *Lancet* 1:1103, 1980.

Obese people consume more fat than lean people:
Swinburn, B. Energy balance or fat balance? *Am J Clin Nutr* 57(suppl):766S, 1993.

Gazzaniga, J. Relationship between diet composition and body fatness, with adjustment for resting energy expenditure and physical activity, in pre-adolescent children. *Am J Clin Nutr* 58:21, 1993.

Blundell, J. Dietary fat and the control of energy intake: evaluating the effects of fat on meal size and postmeal satiety. *Am J Clin Nutr* 57 (suppl): 772S, 1993.

Romieu, I. Energy intake and other determinants of relative weight. *Am J Clin Nutr* 47:406, 1988.

Dreon, D. Dietary fat:carbohydrate ratio and obesity in middle-aged men. *Am J Clin Nutr* 47:995, 1988.

Tremblay, A. Impact of dietary fat content and fat oxidation on energy intake in humans. *Am J Clin Nutr* 49:799, 1989.

Tremblay, A. Nutritional determinants of the increase in energy intake associated with a high-fat diet. *Am J Clin Nutr* 53:1134, 1991.

Prewitt, T. Changes in body weight, body composition, and energy intake in women fed high- and low-fat diets. *Am J Clin Nutr* 54:304, 1991.

Miller, W. Diet composition, energy intake, and nutritional status in relation to obesity in men and women. *Med Sci Sports Exercise* 23:280, 1991.

Chapter 9

Exercise adds to diet therapy:

Gwinup, G. Effect of exercise alone on the weight of obese women. *Arch Intern Med* 135:676: 1975.

Hagen, R. The effects of aerobic conditioning and/or caloric restriction in overweight men and women. *Med Sci Sports Exercise* 18:87, 1986.

Exercise improves mood and self-image:

Daniel, M. Opiate receptor blockade by naltrexone and mood state after acute physical activity. *Br J Sports Med* 26:111, 1992.

Raglin, J. Exercise and mental health. Beneficial and detrimental effects. *Sports Med* 9:323, 1990.

Folkins, C. Physical fitness training and mental health. *Am Psychol* 36:373, 1981.

Carr, D. Physical conditioning facilitates the exercise-induced secretion of beta-endorphins and beta-lipotropin in women. *N Engl J Med* 305:560, 1981.

Exercise relieves depression and anxiety:

Greist, J. Running through your mind. *J Psycho-Somatic Res* 22:259, 1978.

Mersey, D. Health benefits of aerobic exercise. *Postgrad Med* 90:103, 1991.

A high-carbohydrate diet makes things even better: less tension, depression, and anger:

Keith, R. Alterations in dietary carbohydrate, protein, and fat intake and mood state in trained female cyclists. *Med Sci Sports Exercise* 23:212, 1991.

Exercise poses no risk for moderately healthy people:
  Horton, E. Metabolic aspects of exercise and weight reduction. *Med Sci Sports Exercise* 18:10, 1986.

Dietary fat decreases blood oxygen by 20 percent:
  Kuo, P. The effect of lipemia upon coronary circulation and peripheral arterial circulation in patients with essential hyperlipemia. *Am J Med* 26: 68, 1959.

Animal fat makes blood clots, leading to heart attacks:
  Simpson, H. Hypertriglyceridemia and hypercoagulability. *Lancet* 1:786, 1983.
  Ulbright, T. Coronary heart disease: seven dietary factors. *Lancet* 338:985, 1991.

Body uses fat during exercise:
  Rodahl, K. Plasma free fatty acids in exercise. *J Appl Physiol* 19:489, 1964.
  Mole, P. Adaption of muscle to exercise. Increase in levels of palmityl CoA synthetase, carnitine palmityltransferase, and palmityl CoA dehydrogenase, and in the capacity to oxidize fatty acids. *J Clin Invest* 50:2325, 1971.

Postexercise rise in energy expenditure:
  Bielinski, R. Energy metabolism during the postexercise recovery in man. *Am J Clin Nutr* 42:69, 1985.
  Bahr, R. Effect of duration of exercise on excess postexercise O_2 consumption. *J Appl Physiol* 62:485, 1987.
  Brehm, B. Recovery energy expenditure for steady state exercise in runners and nonexercisers. *Med Sci Sports Exercise* 18:205, 1986.

Exercise counteracts plateaus:
  Donahoe, C. Metabolic consequences of dieting and exercise in the treatment of obesity. *J Consult Clin Psychol* 52:827, 1984.

Exercise decreases calorie intake:
  Thompson, J. Exercise and obesity: etiology, physiology, and intervention. *Psych Bull* 91:55, 1982.
  Woo, R. Effect of exercise on spontaneous calorie intake in obesity. *Am J Clin Nutr* 36:470, 1982.
  Woo, R. Voluntary food intake during prolonged exercise in obese women. *Am J Clin Nutr* 36:478, 1982.
  Staten, M. The effect of exercise on food intake in men and women. *Am J Clin Nutr* 53:27, 1991.

Exercise protects muscle during dieting:
  Moyer, C. Body composition changes in obese women on a very low calorie diet with and without exercise. *Med Sci Sports Exercise* 17:292, 1985.

Zuti, B. Comparing diet and exercise as weight reduction tools. *Physician Sports Med* 4:49, 1976.

Three days of exercise a week for fat loss:
Pollock, M. Frequency of training as a determinant for improvement in cardiovascular function and body composition of middle-aged men. *Arch Phys Med Rehabil* 56:141, 1975.
Position Statement on proper and improper weight loss programs. *Med Sci Sports Exercise* 15:ix, 1983.
Dill, D. Oxygen used in horizontal and grade walking and running on the treadmill. *J Appl Physiol* 20:19, 1965.

Exercising at any time is good, but before meals may decrease food intake:
Welle, S. Metabolic responses to a meal during rest and low-intensity exercise. *Am J Clin Nutr* 40:990, 1984.
Greenwood, M. *Obesity.* New York, London, Melbourne: Churchill Livingston, 1983, page 69.

Duration, frequency, and intensity, not type, of exercise are most important:
Pollock, M. Effects of mode of training on cardiovascular function and body composition of adult men. *Med Sci Sports Exercise* 7:139, 1975.

We need 2½ percent of calories as protein:
Rose, W. The amino acid requirements of adult man, XVI, the role of the nitrogen intake. *J Biol Chem* 217:997, 1955.
Hegsted, D. Minimum protein requirements of adults. *Am J Clin Nutr* 21:352, 1968.
Hoffman, W. Nitrogen requirement of normal men on a diet of protein hydrolysate enriched with limiting essential amino acids. *J Nutr* 44:123, 1951.
Dole, V. Dietary treatment of hypertension, clinical and metabolic studies of patients on the Rice-Fruit Diet. *J Clin Invest* 29:1189, 1950.

Spot reduction doesn't work:
Krotkiewski, M. The effect of unilateral isokinetic strength training on local adipose and muscle tissue morphology, thickness, and enzymes. *Eur J Appl Physiol* 42:271, 1979.
Garrow, J. Losing fat. *Lancet* 2:387, 1985.

Chapter 10

Alcohol increases insulin:
Nikkilä, E. Ethanol-induced alterations of glucose tolerance, postglucose hypoglycemia, and insulin secretion in normal, obese, and diabetic subjects. *Diabetes* 24:933, 1975.
Taskinen, M. High density lipoprotein subfractions and postheparin

plasma lipases in alcoholic men before and after ethanol withdrawal. *Metabolism* 31:1168, 1982.

Heavy drinkers are leaner:
Colditz, G. Alcohol intake in relation to diet and obesity in women and men. *Am J Clin Nutr* 54:49, 1991.
Mezey, E. Metabolic impairment and recovery time in acute ethanol intoxication. *J Nerv Mental Dis* 153:445, 1971.

Chocolate, not alcohol, causes weight gain:
Pirola, R. The energy cost of the metabolism of drugs, including ethanol. *Pharmacology* 7:185, 1972.

Alcohol is not turned to fat, but burned as heat:
Lieber, C. Perspectives: Do alcohol calories count? *Am J Clin Nutr* 54:976, 1991.
Lands, W. The case of the missing calories. *Am J Clin Nutr* 54:47, 1991.
Suter, P. The effect of ethanol on fat storage in healthy subjects. *N Engl J Med* 326:983, 1992.

Alcohol replacing carbohydrate results in weight loss:
Pirola, R. The energy cost of the metabolism of drugs, including ethanol. *Pharmacology* 7:185, 1972.

Coffee can cause profound weight loss:
Sours, J. Case reports of anorexia and cafeinism. *Am J Psychiatry* 140:235, 1983.

Caffeine increases metabolic rate, mobilizes fat, causes thermogenesis, and increases respiration:
Higgins, H. The effects of certain drugs on the respiration and gaseous metabolism in normal weight human subjects. *J Pharmacol Exptl Therap* 7:1, 1915.
Acheson, K. Caffeine and coffee: their influence on metabolic rate and substrate utilization in normal and obese individuals. *Am J Clin Nutr* 33:989, 1980.
Jung, R. Caffeine: its effect on catecholamines and metabolism in lean and obese humans. *Clin Sci* 60:527, 1981.

Overweight people drink more coffee:
Haffner, S. Coffee consumption, diet, and lipids. *Am J Epidemiol* 122:1, 1985.
Jacobsen, B. The Tromso Heart Study: The relationship between food habits and the body mass index. *J Chron Dis* 40:795, 1987.

Decaffeinated coffee produces stomach acid:
Cohen, S. Gastric acid secretion and lower-esophageal-sphincter pressure in response to coffee and caffeine. *N Engl J Med* 293:897, 1975.

Ephedrine and caffeine for weight loss:
  Malchow-Moller, A. Ephedrine as an anorectic: the story of the "Elsinore pill." *Int J Obesity* 5:183, 1981.
  Astrup, A. The effect of ephedrine/caffeine mixture on energy expenditure and body composition in obese women. *Metabolism* 41:686, 1992.
  Dulloo, A. The thermogenic properties of ephedrine/methylxanthine mixtures: animal studies. *Am J Clin Nutr* 43:388, 1986.

Chapter 11

High-carbohydrate foods relieve depression:
  Wurtman, J. Effect of nutrient intake on premenopausal depression. *Am J Obstet Gynecol* 161:1228, 1989.

High-carbohydrate foods benefit sleep:
  Philips, F. Isocaloric diet changes and electroencephalographic sleep. *Lancet* 2:723, 1975.

Too much sleep causes mental illness:
  Wehr, T. Improvement of depression and triggering of mania by sleep deprivation. *JAMA* 267:548, 1992.

Sleep control relieves depression:
  Wu, J. The biological basis of an antidepressant response to sleep deprivation and relapse: review and hypothesis. *Am J Psychiatry* 147:14, 1990.
  Leibenluft, E. Is sleep deprivation useful in treatment of depression? *Am J Psychiatry* 149:159, 1992.
  Wu, J. Effect of sleep deprivation on brain metabolism of depressed patients. *Am J Psychiatry* 149:538, 1992.

Chapter 13

High-fat diet impairs circulation:
  Kuo, P. The effect of lipemia upon coronary circulation and peripheral arterial circulation in patients with essential hyperlipemia. *Am J Med* 26:68, 1959.
  Kuo, P. Angina pectoris induced by fat ingestion in patients with coronary artery disease. Ballistocardiographic and electrocardiographic findings. *JAMA* 158:1008, 1955.
  Williams, A. Increased blood agglutination following ingestion of fat, a factor contributing to cardiac ischemia, coronary insufficiency and anginal pain. *Angiology* 8:29, 1957.

Oily skin and hair from your diet:
  Pochi, P. Sebum production, casual sebum levels, titratable acidity of sebum and urinary fractional 17-ketosteroid excretion in males with acne. *J Invest Dermatol* 43:383, 1964.

Wilkinson, D. Psoriasis and dietary fat: The fatty acid composition of surface and scale (ether-soluble) lipids. *J Invest Dermatol* 47:185, 1966.

Acne from a high-fat diet:
Rasmussen, J. Diet and acne (review). *Int J Dermatol* 16:488, 1977.
Rosenberg, E. Acne diet reconsidered. *Arch Dermatol* 117:193, 1981.

Diseases causing skin changes (lupus):
Taylor, H. Systemic lupus erythematosus in Zimbabwe. *Ann Rheum Dis*
45:645, 1986.
Corman, L. The role of diet in animal models of systemic lupus erythematosus: possible implications of human lupus. *Seminars Arthritis Rheum*
15:61, 1985.

Ovarian cysts are common:
Polson, D. Polycystic ovaries—a common finding in normal women. *Lancet*
1:870, 1988.

Diet changes reproductive hormone levels:
Adlercreutz, H. Diet and plasma androgens in postmenopausal vegetarian
and omnivorous women and postmenopausal women with breast cancer. *Am J Clin Nutr* 49:433, 1989.
Woods, M. Low-fat, high-fiber diet and serum estrone sulfate in premenopausal women. *Am J Clin Nutr* 49:1179, 1989.
Rose, D. Effect of a low-fat diet on hormone levels in women with cystic
breast disease. I. Serum steroids and gonadotropins. *J Natl Cancer Inst*
78:623, 1987.
Rose, D. Effect of a low-fat diet on hormone levels in women with cystic
breast disease. II. Serum radioimmunoassayable prolactin and growth
hormone and bioactive lactogenic hormones. *J Natl Cancer Inst* 78:627,
1987.
Howie, B. Dietary and hormonal interrelationships among vegetarian
Seventh-Day Adventists and nonvegetarian men. *Am J Clin Nutr* 42:
127, 1985.
Hill, P. Plasma hormones and lipids in men at different risk of coronary
artery disease. *Am J Clin Nutr* 33:1010, 1980.
Hill, P. Diet, lifestyle and menstrual activity. *Am J Clin Nutr* 33:1192, 1980.
Hill, P. Diet and prolactin release. *Lancet* 2:806, 1976.
Hamalainen, E. Diet and serum sex hormones in healthy men. *J Steroid
Biochem* 20:459, 1984.
Ingram, D. Effect of low-fat diet on female sex hormone levels. *J Natl Cancer
Inst* 79:1225, 1987.
Gorbach, S. Estrogens, breast cancer, and intestinal flora. *Rev Infect Dis*
6(suppl 1):S85, 1984.
Goldin, B. Estrogen excretion patterns and plasma levels in vegetarian and
omnivorous women. *N Engl J Med* 307:1542, 1982.

Goldin, B. Effect of diet on excretion of estrogens in pre- and postmenopausal women. *Ca Res* 41:3771, 1981.
Boyd, N. Effect of a low-fat high-carbohydrate diet on symptoms of cyclical
mastopathy. *Lancet* 2:128, 1988.

High-fat diet contibutes to baldness in men and body hair in women:
Inaba, M. Can human hair grow again? *J Dermatol Surg Oncol* 12:672, 1986.
Conway, G. Hirsutism. *Br Med J* 301:619, 1990.

Body odors from foods:
Cummings, J. Fermentation in the human large intestine: evidence and implications for health. *Lancet* 1:1206, 1983.

Diet causes arterial damage, which causes sexual impotence:
Virag, R. Is impotence an arterial disorder? A study of arterial risk factors
in 440 impotent men. *Lancet* 1:181, 1985.

Medications cause serious sexual dysfunction in 8.3 percent of males:
Curb, J. Long-term surveillance for adverse effects of antihypertensive
drugs. *JAMA* 253:3263, 1985.

Carbohydrate craving and PMS:
Bowen, D. Variations in food preference and consumption across the menstrual cycle. *Physiol Behav* 47:287, 1990.

Chapter 15

Lecithin lowers cholesterol no better than other vegetable fats:
Knuiman, J. Lecithin intake and serum cholesterol. *Am J Clin Nutr* 49:266,
1989.

RECIPE INDEX

GENERAL INDEX

For further information

on Dr. John McDougall's

12-day live-in program,

please call

St. Helena Health Center

at 800-358-9195.

St. Helena Health Center

AT ST. HELENA HOSPITAL

in California's scenic Napa Valley